EAT LIKE A
GODDESS

The Secret Recipe to
End Your Obsession with Food
& Lose Weight Without Trying

Sandy Zeldes

Chef to Celebrities &
Your 'Eat Like a Goddess' Mentor

Sandy Zeldes
P.O. Box 2273
San Rafael, CA 94901
Sandy@EatLikeAGoddess.com
www.EatLikeAGoddess.com

Limits of Liability and Disclaimer of Warranty

Warning – Disclaimer

ISBN-13: 978-1517038793
ISBN-10: 1517038790

Testimonials

ere are some of my clients' stories of success with healing emotional issues, emotional eating, cravings, losing weight, and regaining overall good health, high energy levels, and less body pain as well as creating healthier happier relationships and even making more money or creating new careers while working with me.

Although I cannot guarantee any specific results and the following testimonials do not constitute a warranty or prediction regarding the outcome of someone using EFT or coaching to help end sugar cravings, emotional eating, and dieting, I bring all of my skills and talents to help my clients achieve the best results possible. The following testimonials are what my clients had to say about their own results when working with me.

I Now Have Food Freedom

"I can now make free choices about what I eat and have food freedom. I have let go of so much anger and resentment that it has freed me up to be more loving and kind and present in all my relationships. I have let go of so much self-loathing that it has allowed me to think about what I am capable of beyond just surviving. It has helped me start to feel genuine forgiveness for my parents and look at them more as wounded souls than as monsters. It has helped me forgive myself for the damage I have done to my body with food and for the years I have spent miserable and scared. Because of that, I have started to feel like a grown-up instead of a wounded child, which has allowed me to make choices about what I eat and how I treat myself and how I allow others to treat me. I can act instead of react. I don't have to react out of fear. I can take my time and decide what the next step is. I think that if I had gotten even one of the things listed above out of our work together, I would be satisfied, so to get all of them, makes me feel truly blessed and grateful.

Sharon

I Feel Lighter, Freer & Open to Possibility

"I've never felt this much of a change and I've worked with all kinds of energy healers and other EFT practitioners. This is really different. I can really feel the difference. I feel lighter, freer, open to so much more possibility and the neat thing is that I don't feel a dependency on you like you have to do it for me. You give me lots of tools I can use for myself and I feel like my own best healer. I so respect you and I love you so much. It's about everything, not just about the food. It's about my life, my vision, living my dreams. THANK YOU."

Danielle

Lost the Weight & Love Looking in the Mirror

"I can't believe how scared I was to get started working with you. I simply didn't believe that I could be successful at this when I hadn't been in the past but that is EXACTLY why I was successful this time I think because this was so different than anything I'd tried before. I'd been focused on all the wrong things maybe. When I tapped for everything but the food it all turned around for me. I had out of control cravings when we started and now they are at a ZERO, even when I'm upset! I'm consistently losing weight not from a 'diet' but from eating the way I need to that feels right to me. I'm not obsessing much or thinking about it, it's just coming off. But best of all I'm refocused on what is important to me in my life. I feel very positive instead of in a downward spiral with negative thinking. I even had this really bad victim way of thinking and the past kept repeating itself. Not anymore. I'm handling situations that would have totally thrown me off before, with a lot more ease. I'm looking forward to what comes next instead of fearing moving forward in my life. My confidence is so much higher now, I can't wait. Thank you so much!"

Kalena

Stopped Focusing on Food

"I never thought it would really be possible for me to STOP focusing on food… but I HAVE. I always thought there would have to be a charge around food, or it would always be difficult but I would just get better at handling it. That was my goal. When you said 'no, it doesn't have to be this way at all' I didn't believe it, but now, after working with you, I can have something and not feel guilty about it and food just isn't an issue in my life. I don't spend my whole day focused on thinking about food, I think about ok, what is next for me. Which is my dreams and my business and how I was holding myself back in a MAJOR way. Now I'm in action, I'm doing it and in a way that works for me."

Elizabeth

My Stomach Is Flatter After Our First Session

"I wanted to talk to you right after we worked together to tell you that my stomach is already flatter…Everything in my life is better, I just had the best day of my life. I was excited like a little kid. It was awesome. Did we really just clear this blockage? Anyways I feel good, so thank you so much."

Heather

No More Making Myself Sick with Cookie Dough!

"Friday was a big day for me – 'twas my annual cookie baking day. In years past, I would've made myself sick with dough and cookies but this year was completely different. There was no frenzy around needing to taste the dough or shove cookies in. I was super calm and almost subdued. So whatever work we've done has had an impact – and I'm woot-wooting all over the place!"

Stacey V

I Lost 10 Pounds Without Cravings or Hunger!

"I was so exhausted I couldn't exercise and felt I couldn't seem to take action; I was too busy. I also struggled with emotional eating my whole life and had no control over sugar cravings. Whenever there was emotional instability I would eat emotionally. I also had a hard time making healthy choices or being balanced with food. After around four weeks I now have lost 10 lbs. and am not eating emotionally! I'm making healthy choices because I want to and best of all I am no longer tired all the time, am exercising regularly and have lots of energy!"

Jennifer Molloy

Lost 10 Pounds with Less Obsession About Food

"After working with Sandy, I feel much more supported, less all alone, am experiencing a greatly improved relationship with my husband, much better boundaries with my mom, am eating cleaner, and resisting that less. I have much more of a desire to nurture myself with food instead of rebelling and taking things out on myself with negative eating patterns. After 27 years of this food disorder and struggle, I am relieved to have less of a grip for the need for food. I am calm and relaxed more and when not feeling that way, have lots of tools that work for me. I am listening to my needs and myself now more. My binging and obsessing about food has decreased dramatically. When I fall off the eating that is best for my body, it can be hard to get back on, but I do. The instances where I fall off are rarer. I am more proactive with meal planning and it doesn't feel impossible now like it did before. I am much less negative about how I am thinking about food. I no longer feel I have to hurt myself this way with food. I've lost 10 lbs. and some of the bloating, which made me feel much better about myself and how I look in my clothes. Thanks, Sandy!"

T.G.

Lost 1½ sizes

"In the last three months of working with you I've lost 1½ clothing sizes. I'm so much more inspired and energized. Difficult work situations that stressed me out no longer do—and nobody there has changed, but I have changed how I feel! What is great about working with you is that you really go get what is the real deal inside and get quickly into the core of the problem. The layers are peeled away one by one to find that things are really as simple as you can think they should be. I find it fantastic how you can go in on my energy and ask what the problem really is. I feel enlightened and more aware of what my issues really are. I find it mysterious when you release the different things that have been built up. I feel much better since I have worked with you and realize that all my problems are self-made because of the built up of walls of protection since my childhood. I am looking forward to doing so much more work with you and progress into a better being for myself and the people who surround me. I am very happy to have met you. Oh, and by the way, as a side benefit of all the emotional clearing work, my 20-year problem with back pain is gone!"

C.W.

Energy & Confidence Back Almost Overnight!

"When I first started working with Sandy only two months ago I was barely able to get through the day I had such low energy and a hard time focusing. I also struggled with anxiety, was very sensitive emotionally (which I thought was just my personality) and food cravings. I took a lot of naps and couldn't get a lot of work done, it seemed, without being exhausted. I also felt a lack of confidence in client relationships. Working out even mildly would wipe me out. In fact in our first session, I could hardly stay on the phone I was so tired. But after implementing even the first few things that Sandy recommended I was feeling much, much better, even the next day! It was amazing. Though there were ups and downs as I was recovering, I began to have my energy back more and more with time. I now can work out without wiping myself out, my clear thinking is back. I feel more confident, even in client relationships, less obsessive and anxious, don't have food cravings and feel like I did many years ago and my energy is consistently strong throughout the day. In fact I started bringing in big clients during the time I was working with Sandy and I had the energy and confidence to do it! I am so grateful for the support I've received from you… it's made a big difference for me. I was beginning to feel hopeless. I'm referring a few friends to you."

Lynn Rousseau

Sugar Cravings & Fatigue Decreased Dramatically

"Sandy is like a walking encyclopedia when it comes to health! I described my symptoms of sugar cravings, excess weight and fatigue, and she was quick to recommend what she thought would help. And her recommendations worked! Within just a few weeks, most of my symptoms had disappeared! I highly recommend Sandy if you want help with improving your energy, health and well-being."

Sonika T.

Stopped Binging on Ice Cream & Bread

"It's a victory to not eat a half gallon of ice cream at night and the bread all day etc. that I binge on. All my life I've been doing this and now it's just gone without even trying. I don't force myself, I just don't want it. I don't even think about it. And I've lost a few pounds—all in just a few weeks of working with you. Yay!"

T.G.

I've Slimmed Down in Just a Few Weeks

"I feel a big difference in my stress level. Before I was so constricted and tense and unable to relax at all. This is a very big difference for me to be able to relax at work and in my life even when things are crazy around me. My mind isn't going like a maniac all the time! And I've slimmed down a lot! I feel great. After just a few works of working together I've achieved what I've never achieved before. Thank you."

C.W.

Food Obsession & Body Hatred Gone

"I wanted you to know that I have totally stopped thinking about food obsessively AT ALL. It's not even a thought in my mind. I'm not obsessed, I have no cravings, I'm not over-eating; it's just gone!! It's been three weeks or more and nothing. The 'evil me' who hates and criticizes my body constantly—gone!! I am sleeping well, feel great, and don't think about food like I used to constantly. This is amazing. And it was easy. I didn't have to force anything. This problem I've had for years now is gone."

Seilya

I Don't Even Think About Food at All Now!

"I've stopped thinking about food obsessively at all... no nighttime or dinnertime eating issues. I was able to completely stop eating or craving wheat without even trying, and it's only been a few weeks. I accomplished all of this without even having to try or think about it. Amazing. I was struggling with exercising (you know it was on my 'to do' list for forever), and now last week I exercised every day and enjoyed it! This is exciting progress and in such a short time. I'm really excited."

Dianne

I've lost 7½ lbs. in the last two weeks effortlessly!

"It has only been less than two weeks and I've lost 7½ lbs. without even trying. This has never happened before. I'm sleeping better without really trying anything new, my energy is MUCH BETTER—I straightened out a counter top that has been literally cluttered since I can't remember—and I feel better than I have in a long time…like my old self again. Thank you so much!"

L.L.

Low Energy, Difficulty Focusing & Emotional Sensitivity Gone!

"Before starting to work with Sandy I suffered from severe allergies, anxiety, cravings for sweets and salty foods, and mood swings. I also had very low energy and difficulty focusing on what I needed to do and felt very emotionally sensitive. To top it off I had started getting acid reflux! I no longer suffer from just about all of these symptoms, definitely not to the degree that I did only three months ago, and in fact have gotten off of both my allergy and reflux medication! I am working out more and feeling more motivated as well. Thank you, Sandy!

"I recommend Sandy highly!"

Kristi A.

I Ended the Habit of Emotional Eating

"I found Sandy on a web search because I knew I needed help. My emotional eating was spinning out of control (chocolate bar, ice cream, and cookies every day) and I had gained 35 pounds (and I'm only 5'2"). I was very low energy and depressed as my mom was diagnosed with stage 4 cancer and died less than three months later. I had daily sugar cravings and insomnia off and on. I'd worked with therapists, nutritionists, and personal trainers; read Geneen Roth's books; and even went to one of her workshops out of town. None of it worked. Now if someone told me my cravings and binges would end in one month after working with Sandy I would've said it was impossible. But after four weeks of working with Sandy, the cravings were gone (physical cravings). And then we worked on changing my behavior as well so that not only were my physical cravings gone, but I ended the habit of emotional eating. My energy has returned and my depression has lifted and now I regularly exercise four to six times a week. I have a renewed vitality and zest for life and I'm feeling better than ever. I give Sandy my highest recommendation!"

Tamara

I've lost 8 pounds—over Christmas!

"I lost a few pounds (8 pounds), and that in Christmas season in Germany, not bad at all. I didn't starve, just ate in the way I have applied since our first calls…and it works!

"Thank you, Sandy!"

Josanne Holland

Depression, Low Energy, Anxiety & Sleeplessness All Gone

"Thanks Sandy! I've been really, really happy with how working with you is going! My skin is radiant now. I have more energy, motivation, drive, and determination to achieve the goals I set out for myself.

"You know, it's hard for me to even remember how I was feeling just a few months ago, I feel so different now. It's hard to relate to it. I feel really, really good. It's amazing. Just two months ago when I started sessions with you I was extremely depressed, and had been crying basically daily for a few years. I was worried that I had no motivation, my energy was low, and I was having some anxiety and sleeplessness problems at times. I've wanted to lose some weight also for a while but didn't really have the drive to do anything about it. Now I'm registered for a half marathon, doing yoga, sleeping well, not crying at all or feeling depressed at all, excited about my life, and have so many creative projects I'm working on. I would say every single thing I began sessions to work on are well on their way to being accomplished now. That is really amazing. Thanks, Sandy. I really appreciate this. You are really great at what you do! All of this and it's just two months into my program!

"I highly to recommend working with you! I want to spread the word."

Megan E.

Lost 18 Pounds & Feeling Great!
P.S. Six Months Later & Have Lost 60 Pounds!

"Before I worked with Sandy I had a lot of trouble with cravings and binging on comfort foods and I was at my highest weight and depressed about that. Now I can tell that I'm handling emotions better and everything else better. I'm able to take action in a way that works for me toward my goals now instead of struggling. I feel differently too, like if I'm unhappy looking in the mirror, I really get it that I need to take care of myself now. I actually WANT to now. I am feeling more able to take positive healthy steps that work for me with my health and weight. I think now 'I'm hungry. I need nourishment,' and I give myself what I need instead of eating my favorite comfort foods. I'm getting more comfort now out of eating healthy foods than the old comfort foods.

"I also used to rely a lot on what others I admired would tell me was 'right' to eat, and now I listen to my own body and follow that instead, and it works. I know there is no other authority higher than myself.

"And I've lost 18 pounds and I'm feeling GREAT! I'm motivated and it feels really good."

Less than six months later Terri sent me this about her success with weight loss as well, and she wanted to add this to her testimonial above.

"P.S.: We haven't even discussed weight loss in a long time! The thing I originally told you was the most important thing for me to work on—and we haven't even mentioned it in the longest time! I haven't missed it! I feel that my diet is about health and that I am always willing to consider the possibility of even healthier options. I feel very in control. I have actively been making effort toward eating healthy and taking the excess weight off. I've gone through several holidays and birthdays and other food events. At all of these events I have eaten as I wished, felt great, and was perfectly happy to flow easily back in to my general eating plan without any rebounding or cravings after the events were over. This stuff would have been my usual sabotage as, until now, I was not able to 'eat a little bit bad' sometimes and 'super strict' other times; it had to be all or nothing. If I swayed, I swayed far and that made me afraid to ever sway and that made me sad and weird. **Thank you for helping me to have this control over food. This has brought me sanity and the ability to enjoy food again. To date I have taken off 60 lbs.!** I still have more that I will be taking off. I know that I will get there and, this time, stay there!!!"

Terri S.

Struggle with Food & Sugar Cravings Vanished!

"Sandy has been tireless in helping me with my issues. Her enthusiasm and determination on my behalf have been so inspiring and have helped me to stay focused on my goals when I would otherwise have given up. My out-of-control sugar cravings are now gone, and my energy level is really great now. I highly recommend Sandy."

Alison W.

A Lifetime of Sugar Cravings & Self-Criticism--Disappeared!

"By the end of just a few sessions I was very excited and surprised to realize I was NOT getting sick, which was a first, while being under a lot of stress with work. Sandy has helped me start to untangle the web of self-criticism and stress, and she has done it with sensitivity, skill, and good humor. Besides helping me with painful emotions, she has helped considerably to curb this client's lifetime addiction to sweets and in a matter of days no less! This is really amazing. I'm not eating the ice cream at night even after just beginning to implement the few dietary changes you recommended. After just 1 week I noticed that my cravings had stopped, and it continued into the third week as well. I'm feeling steady energy and not snacking, either. This is really new for me. Three months out, still feeling amazing and no cravings!"

Cindy R.

Motivation & Energy Return; Depression Lifts

"When I contacted Sandy I was in what I think is my rock bottom and was very depressed. My sister had just died, and I'd gained weight and I was having a really hard time getting back into working out. I was feeling tired and unmotivated. After only three sessions, I've started exercising and I'm not so tired anymore and I feel hopeful now that I am going to be ok. I know that I am on my way to feeling better every day, and though I am still sad about what happened, I no longer feel depressed. I highly recommend Sandy."

Suzanne K.

Cravings for Snacks, Sweets 7 Wine Disappeared

"I can't believe that I'm just not even thinking about having my wine or favorite snacks at night now. And we didn't even talk about taking those things away. I'm just not needing them anymore. Amazing. I feel MUCH more energetic and get through the day better now too. Thanks Sandy. I look forward to working with you again soon!"

Danielle K.

Acknowledgments & Dedication

This book is dedicated to my grandmother, my mother, my sister, and my beautiful niece, Hana. All of you in your own way have been an inspiration to me.

My grandmother, for providing some of my first memories of home-cooked meals and long leisurely dinner times with family. I still can recall the smells coming from her kitchen with love.

My mother, for being a friend and a mentor on the road to health, sustainable living, and my current accelerated spiritual practice since she passed away in 2008. Thank you, Mom, for showing me that love is the answer now and forever, no matter the question, and is all there is. Your presence ignites and inspires me still.

My sister, for her strength and courage and for showing me that anything is possible.

My niece, for bringing so much joy into my life.

This book is also dedicated to preserving, respecting, and nurturing a balanced relationship to the natural environment.

I can think of nothing that has truly inspired me more urgently than a desire to be of service in healing this relationship that we as a world community have so deeply wounded.

If there is a mission behind what I have worked so hard to learn and then teach it is to inspire joy and love for ourselves first to the point that we then take that into the world and create the balance with the Earth that we so desperately need at this time.

When we truly love and are compassionate with ourselves I feel we become the change we wish to see in the world. Often being loving and compassionate with ourselves really begin with our relationship with food as women, and this relationship with food is foundational to healing the Earth at this time.

My heartfelt appreciation goes out to all of the women who have inspired me that I've worked with who have literally altered the course of their lives and found not only peace but true happiness and joy in their lives, no matter what the situation was when we first began working together.

You have been a real inspiration to me, and I am honored to have been a part of your path.

Deep bow.

This book is also dedicated to all of you, and for those of you yet to find your total goddess transformation!

Welcome. You are a Goddess now and forever.

Blessings and joy,

~ **Sandy**

Your "Eat Like a Goddess" Mentor

Get Your
Free Companion Audio &
Resource Guide Here!

"Insider Tips From
Your Eat Like a Goddess Mentor:
How to End Food Obsession & Love Yourself Skinny"

If you've struggled with diets that don't work, and you just want to love how you look in the mirror and feel like the goddess that you truly are and don't want to feel deprived to lose weight, I invite you to get your Eat Like a Goddess Support Package, featuring top-selling course author on the popular website Daily Om and chef to many high-profile celebrities and business leaders, Sandy Zeldes.

In this free audio program you will learn:

- **The Invisible Three**: Identify and release the three invisible barriers that keep you locked in a never-ending battle with food, weight, and your body.

- **Get Clear on the Cause**: Why weight is not the issue, food is not your enemy, and how to clear the root cause of those extra pounds.

- **A New Breakthrough!** A revolutionary process that makes is super-easy for you to clear hidden obstacles to losing weight.

- **Why Willpower Doesn't Work**: The real truth about willpower, dieting, and exercise, and why any kind of force or effort simply won't work.

- **The Deal Breaker**: The most important truth you must know if you are to ever change your relationship with food and your body.

- **Cut the Cravings**: The quickest way to retrain your brain so you no longer have the slightest craving or interest in certain foods.

- **Fall in Love**: How to relax into a sweet and loving relationship with your body and food, forever.

Don't Waste One More Second Obsessing About Food or Your Weight! You Know You Were Meant for So Much More!

No more diets. No more being jerked around by food or cravings. No more binge eating or reaching for those comfort foods any time you feel emotional or tired.

Stop wasting your precious time and energy focusing on food and your body weight! This is about you taking your life back so you can have more of who you really are, **more energy, more love, more joy**.

But best of all, you can release food obsession and lose weight with these tools with *__much less effort__*!

Take the next step and sign up for your Eat Like a Goddess Support Package, a $97 value and yours FREE, my gift to you, full of rich information gathered over years of working with women to transform their relationship to food so that they can eat and feel like the goddess that they truly are.

Get Your Free Companion Audio & Resource Guide Here

www.EatLikeAGoddess.com

About Sandy Zeldes

Sandy Zeldes grew up in a food-loving family where she developed much appreciation for food, cooking and eating. An old family story goes that as everyone was gathered around the table for dinner one evening with her grandparents, as a young 6-year-old Sandy got all choked up and began crying as she told her grandmother that when she died all Sandy wanted were her recipes!

This was just the beginning of a massive love affair with food, cooking, eating, obsessing and learning about what to eat and how to cook. Fast forward twenty years and she created Sandy's Gourmet Productions, a private chef and catering company born out of a desire to provide gourmet cuisine for a specialized market in Hawaii, where Sandy resided from 1992 to 2002.

After graduating from the University of California at Berkeley with a bachelor's degree in Anthropology, Sandy went to Hawaii for a 'vacation', planning to return to the Bay Area and pursue a graduate degree in Public Health... but her love of being in the kitchen and playing with food took over and she started a private chef and catering business in Hawaii.

Meanwhile, Sandy's cravings and food obsession followed and plagued her in her 20's until she became a Certified Nutrition Consultant and had a massive paradigm shift. Her breakthrough? Eat what actually nurtured her instead of a dietary dogma that had developed in her life. That was the first step, followed by putting it into action consistently—without having to use willpower.

As a chef, rebel nutritionist and wildly passionate food lover, Sandy found the final missing link with using Emotional Freedom Techniques (EFT) along with other stress relief and energy healing techniques. The result? Eating became as joyful again as when she sat at the table when she was 6 years old crying with happiness over the love of her grandmother's cooking.

And now Sandy is sharing these secrets with her clients— and with you!

By the way, Sandy's clients are as diverse as high profile celebrities, business and marketing industry leaders, health retreat leaders, coaches, entrepreneurs, professional performers and stay-at-home moms.

Many of the women Sandy works with are extremely successful in different areas of their lives and yet often still struggle with food. They want to stop beating themselves up about it and instead have more confidence and feel naturally motivated to eat healthily.

Sandy is the author of the best selling course on Daily Om: Healing Subconscious Blocks to Weight Loss, which was number 1 on its bestseller list for more than 8 weeks when it was released in 2012. Sandy has featured on EFT.net, EFT Universe, The Tapping Solution Energy Psychology online, and *Elephant Journal*. She has also appeared on NBC, Fox News, ABC, CBS, *The Wall Street Journal* and *The San Francisco Chronicle*.

Sandy's Story:

How a Chef to Celebrities Finds the Secret to End Dieting, Emotional Eating, and Poor Body Image

used to have a love-hate relationship with food. You could even say that I was in an abusive relationship with the stuff. One minute I would be in heaven eating the best meal in the world, but then the next minute hating myself for, well, eating at all.

Had I eaten too much?

Had I eaten "wrong" or "bad" foods?

Should I be eating a vegan, vegetarian, raw, or another diet?

Maybe a high-protein or low-carb diet?

How much fat, protein, and carbohydrate should I eat, and which kinds?

Which diet was right?

It was enough to make me crazy, and feel guilty all the time with food.

I would also work out like crazy.

I used to think that if I couldn't do a two-hour run, even when I was already in pain from the previous day's work out and feeling exhausted, I hadn't done enough of a workout!

I actually feel sick to my stomach just thinking about it now. I made myself sick then, too. Literally.

I often hated my body because it didn't conform to an image I believed I had to be. Even at my lowest weight I thought I was fat. I had to ask myself:

What good is becoming thin if I won't love myself or be happy at that *weight?*

Nothing really changed because I kept trying the same things over and over.

I didn't know then what I know now.

The years rolled by and as I continued to try different diets and work out like crazy, I'd have periods of giving up that would last a year or two here or there where I'd gain 10 to 15 pounds and say, "Screw it. It's all BS. I may as well go wild and eat all I want and not exercise at all!"

But then I'd be back in the same place where I started: begging to feel good and most of all wanting it to feel easier to be at a healthy weight.

Damn those skinny friends who never had this problem! They didn't even seem to have to work out. How irritating!

We all know a few.

Guess what their secret is?

It isn't a secret! They are doing exactly what you see them doing: nothing.

Okay, well maybe not nothing. But close. *That is the point.*

They aren't destroying their metabolism by *not* eating, or eating too little, or working out so hard they almost kill themselves—and they don't seem to suffer from severe self-criticism.

Unfair? Well, at first glance it seems to be.

But when you peel away the layers you realize that you can be like them.

It really is possible to do less, eat more, and feel better, sexier, healthier, and more energized *without* dieting!

For many years I was a sought-after professional chef to high-profile celebrities, and during that time I was one of the most health-conscious people I knew, too—eating loads of organic, local vegetables and whole grains. In fact, as a professional chef I mostly cooked for myself, too. I was constantly studying health and nutrition. I went to conferences, I read every popular book, I even became obsessed with nutritional supplements and whole-food supplements way before any of that was popular. Trust me: It wasn't easy to talk about green foods and green powders in the 1990s.

One of the biggest turning points for me was in the process of becoming a chef over the years beginning in 1993 and learning how to cook meals that nourished my body and soul. I thought I was pretty healthy. In fact, I looked it, too.

How frustrating that even after all of that I couldn't seem to control my cravings, felt bloated half the time when I ate, and had all manner of health concerns from insomnia to uterine fibroids and excruciatingly painful periods. (I went to the emergency room a few times for the pain. Some of you can relate to this.)

It was only after I decided to make a career out of nutrition and went back to school to take a holistic health two-year-long certification program in 2005 that I began to see what was missing in my "perfect" picture of healthy eating.

I learned some amazing things about improving my health that left me astounded by how much better I felt when I applied them.

The secret I discovered was the opposite of what I thought I would discover. The secret was not taking any foods out of my diet, nor being restrictive, but adding amazingly tasty foods in. Deprivation was never the answer.

I learned that you not only can eat like a goddess, but you must to regain your health and kick sugar cravings.

You would think all this great information would have been enough to change it all, right?

Wrong!

I had all of this great new information about health and what to eat to feel great, but I couldn't always put it into action. This is the second-most-common problem so many people have—right after not knowing what to eat that works for them uniquely and getting confused by all the conflicting diet advice out there.

We struggle at times to actually do what we know will make us feel our best. We come home exhausted or stressed and end up in the fridge looking for comfort. Or maybe we are so stressed at work that we grind down on loads of junk food and don't even know what happened. I've heard that one a lot from clients: "I just can't avoid the candy dish (or pastries and sweets) at work." I understand. I know. I get it. I've been there. The good news is you can change this without using willpower.

Half of the solution is knowing what to eat that works best for us as individuals, and the other half of the solution is putting this knowledge into action!

At about the same time that I was learning so much about nutrition that just rocked my world (and totally shocked my world, too), I began learning about a method to release stress and emotions. It was EFT: Emotional Freedom Techniques. It was a few years later that I pursued a certification in the technique and began using it effectively with clients.

Effective, expert use of EFT and other emotional release and healing techniques combined with nutrition began to change everything with food, cravings, weight, and body image once and for all for me—and later for my clients. The knowledge of what to eat and then being able to take action with ease instead of force and helping people let go of self-sabotage became a powerful solution to an overwhelming problem.

Many of my clients went from having a lifelong love/hate relationship with food and their bodies; poor body image, low energy and extreme fatigue; debilitating low self-esteem; lack of motivation to exercise or eat healthy; being overweight, stressed, and anxious; having out-of-control food cravings; binge eating; and feeling like a total failure to feeling super confident, happy, and joyful in their own skin; having peace with food and their bodies; being free from food and sugar cravings, food obsession, and binge eating; and free from chronic dieting and the yo-yo that comes with it of weight gain to being able to create peace with food and their bodies. This gave them so much more than that as well. Relationships blossomed, both work related and personal. Financial and creative pursuits blossomed for almost all of them as well. It has been truly inspiring to watch as healing this issue touched their whole lives.

For more information about me you can visit my website: www.EatLikeAGoddess.com/about.

Is This Book for Me?

"Instead of giving myself reasons why I can't,
I give myself reasons why I can."
~ *Unknown*

As a savvy woman you probably already are well aware of the benefits of a healthy diet, emotional well-being, and having balance in your life. Physical and mental health are significant contributions to living a full and meaningful life, right? If you are like all of my clients, the problem becomes *doing* the things we know we have to to stay healthy and balanced. There is an information overload out there and a plethora of new, hip diets. I like to joke sometimes that my clients know more about diet trends than I do as a chef and nutritionist! In fact, many would definitely call it an obsession of theirs to try each and every new trend. Unfortunately, this doesn't get them the results that they seek, or it would be great to have all this knowledge.

So what is really going on?

If you are like the vast majority of people on a diet there is one agonizing problem with dieting: It doesn't work! You can gain and lose the same weight over and over again, creating a new problem: hopelessness.

What if the problem isn't an inability to lose weight but an inability to continue on a rigorous and rigid diet plan that sucks?

What if the problem is truly in the underlying way of

approaching the whole problem in the first place? And now let me ask you the ultimate crazy question: What if there is no problem, but focusing on the "problem" actually is creating it?

I know. It probably doesn't even make sense right now to hear that, but I'm telling you: The problem is definitely not the problem. We have created it.

Here is how it works.

Chronic food obsession or caloric restriction creates binges and weight concerns if it is a long-term issue. We start out excited and hopeful, fasting on juices and smoothies or paleo madness, and what happens?

Do you make it past three weeks? Maybe you make it three months, as many of my clients do, and then the backslide happens into binges. And the binges are equal in their intensity as the restriction or worse.

Then there are those stressful moments at the end of the day, or when the kids come home, or at work when someone pisses you off. What happens then? Does the cookie dough, doughnuts, or that little bowl of candies left out call to you and you can't stop?

You would not be alone if so. Comfort foods are naturally the very foods that are also sweet or carbohydrate rich.

So is the problem the food? Is it the diet? Is it the binges? Maybe it is the stress?

It is none of those things.

You see, for the women who come to me who have struggled with cravings, emotional eating habits, and food obsessions, there is this other problem that, when addressed, eliminates the need to focus on the food at all.

There is no lack of information here. Most of my clients, as I said, could teach a course on holistic nutrition, vitamins, and supplements, and know about stress-relief techniques. They have gym and yoga memberships. They are often self-proclaimed "spiritual" or self-aware, and very savvy professionals and moms.

The only problem is actually a very simple one: They are

shooting an arrow at the *wrong* target. They are getting a bull's-eye, but it is literally at the wrong target.

Their body is not the problem, and neither is food.

There is an underlying cause and it is within us. This is not about blame or shame here, let me be clear. But this should reassure you, since it puts all of the power right back in your hands. This is a very positive thing.

Now we just have to shoot the arrow at the *right* target and move forward.

What is the right target? This is the focus of this book. The right target for someone struggling with food obsessions or emotional eating, or who feels constantly deprived with dieting, is to address emotional stress that may have accumulated in their lives and beliefs around food and their bodies that sabotage results.

If you are health conscious or have tried so many diets that you can't name them all but still struggle with debilitating health concerns and weight gain, you will love this approach.

If you tend to get down on yourself constantly and wonder if, with all you know, you should have been able to control over-eating and cravings, you are definitely in the right place.

If you're like many of the women I talk with, you also feel sick of constantly feeling self-conscious in your body and tired of not being able to wear the clothes you want to wear, and can't stick to a diet because the cravings are out of control, and no matter what they do they can't get a handle on it. They feel exhausted and sometimes hopeless about ever being able to get this under control, and the fear of diabetes, heart disease, or even cancer lurks in the back of their minds. But, maybe even worse, they often feel like their weight or this problem with food is holding them back in some way from doing what they want to in life or living fully. I have found that there is also a recurring theme of feeling like a failure, no matter what else they have achieved in life (and many, if not most, of the women who contact me are extremely successful) because they have failed at either losing weight or ending emotional eating.

Knowing what to eat that works for you as an individual, and being able to stick to what you know *without having to use willpower or force* are the first steps to finding peace with food and your body, lose weight naturally, and have optimal health.

In this book I will show you how to do both.

Possible Roadblocks to Success

If you have tried to lose weight and end cravings or emotional eating, you know there can be problems that can stop you in your tracks.

Here are a few things that I see can be stopping people:

There is conflicting (and confusing) health information out there.

Maybe you've read every book about health and tried every diet from Atkins to raw foods diets to cleanses. Maybe you've had some success and felt better at times, and then struggled with cravings even though you thought you were doing everything that was taught.

You might have started to feel like you have no idea how to decipher all the conflicting information and given up!

What I have discovered is that the secrets to lasting weight loss have nothing to do with food for so many people. If you struggle with cravings, emotional eating, stress eating, self-sabotage, or not being able to do what you feel you know you need to, the answers are somewhere other than with the food first before looking at what diet is "right" for you.

Some of the diet confusion that exists can be due to an inability to hear our own inner wisdom after being at war with food and our bodies for so long. When we let go of the inner struggles we tend to drop our addictive habits and move forward, knowing what is uniquely right for us as an individual.

I don't have the time or energy.

One thing that I have noticed over time is that we, as women, often prioritize everyone else's needs over our own needs. Often prioritizing our own health and well-being is essential before we can recover our energy and begin to stop being overwhelmed.

Sometimes that is truly the first step in healing. In saying no to others, extra commitments, and putting too much on our schedules, we say yes to ourselves. This is extremely nourishing and empowering. We create time for what we value most. Do we value ourselves? What can you say no to, so that you can say yes to yourself now? Asking for support from others is another way to create time and get out of overwhelm so you can begin to make yourself and your own needs a priority. Finding ways to get that support is often an important first step.

It will be too expensive.

Yes, there is a financial investment often in getting our health back, but I have to ask you: What will you do without your health? How much do health issues like diabetes, cancer, heart disease, high blood pressure, and other major health concerns cost people in our country? All are partially preventable through simply taking better care of ourselves.

I recently had a client tell me how expensive her "junk food" habit was. She estimated that she was spending *double* every month in food costs because of it. I wonder sometimes how much all those extra foods cost.

Honestly, though, the ultimate cost cannot even be determined financially, but in a life not lived for many. What is the cost of not having the confidence or energy to start that new business, go on a date, have healthier relationships in general, or desire to be social because of feeling lousy all the time?

I don't trust myself to be able to follow through.

The keys to success with any program are follow-through, being able to take consistent action, and staying focused.

The key to being able be consistent is to get out of our own way sometimes. However, the motivation is there in the beginning but is only temporarily for many people. Why is this?

In short, we get into self-sabotage often the minute we set out on achieving an important goal.

When we sabotage ourselves, or feel lazy or unmotivated, there is always a good reason for our actions (or lack of actions), but they are often out of our conscious awareness.

Discovering our subconscious motivations and reasons for our behaviors is where change and action really start to happen for many.

So if you've been struggling with being able to follow through with a plan of action for a long time and don't understand why, you are in good company. It is actually quite normal, and learning what is going on for us within is where the magic lies to creating the change we wish to see.

I like to use the analogy of driving down the road with our foot on both the gas and the brake at the same time. That is what it is like to have a goal but feel like we can't stay motivated long enough to stay in action.

Many of you probably know how to drive down the road already. You know what to eat primarily that works for you, and you have a sense of what you need to do, but you can't seem to do it consistently. The brake is whatever is making the food so compelling right now that it is no longer a choice but an obsession. Having the brakes on also looks like lack of motivation to get into action in many different ways that would help you achieve your goal. All you need to do is figure out how to get your foot off of the brake, which is the purpose of this book and the work that I do with my clients daily.

If this describes you right now, you're in good company, as I've said.

There is a reason that dieting and weight loss is a multi-billion-dollar industry in the United States alone. However, the answer is not in another diet or better exercise program.

I've tried before and failed, so why would this be any different?

The secrets to lasting weight loss have nothing at all whatsoever to do with food. All of the secrets to lasting weight loss are within *you.*

In this book I will help you discover these secrets. I've got your back, Goddess. We're going to walk through a process that all of my most successful clients have implemented and that I myself have used to heal a lifelong obsession with food.

The reason this particular approach is so different is because it is not "one size fits all" and looking at all of the external things to do that you probably have already tried before. The reason this is different and actually stands a chance is because it is about *you* and why the weight and food habits make perfect sense. When we address our true motivations, often subconsciously we are shooting the arrow at the right target —and actually hitting our mark.

You see, it isn't that any one diet or exercise program is wrong or right. It's just that when we focus on that as the "problem" to be solved we are simply looking in the wrong place for the answer.

Believe in yourself. Believe that you deserve to have compassion for yourself now. If you can do that and do it now, you are on your way already to lasting peace with food.

The Dalai Lama has said that compassion is love in action.

Love is a verb, my friend. There is no time like the present to get started with giving that love and compassion to yourself. In so doing, we find the true answers we seek, food is no longer the enemy, and our bodies are perfect just the way they are. From this place we tend to make much better choices that bring us back into balance with weight and overall health and well-being.

Contents

Introduction

n this book I will not be telling you what you can or cannot do. Reasons for this are many. Many people have already heard repeatedly what *not* to do, and I think that sets them up for feeling deprived, and ultimately like a failure when they can't stick to a rigid plan after a while.

To get results I approach things from a different angle.

I want you to feel inspired, excited, motivated naturally instead of through force and willpower, energized, and hopeful.

The women I have worked with over the years knew what to do and could practically teach a course on nutrition! They were simply beat down with new diets and information telling them what they can and can't do. The only trouble was they couldn't follow it.

That's a problem, isn't it?

It's the number-one problem I focus on with the information in this book. So if you have tried everything and failed, you are in the right place. It's time to face in a new direction.

The basic foundational insider strategies are truly all you need to get started *now* toward optimal health and face in that new direction. The strategies are twofold: nutritional and emotional.

The nutritional strategies offered can make a significant difference fast with cravings and weight loss without dieting or taking any foods away. In fact, I highly recommend that you do not eliminate any foods unless you really want to. If it feels natural to, then great—do it. But the whole point is to help you find what feels natural to you based on what you desire from a place of deep awareness and knowing of what works for you as an individual—not a "one size fits all" diet—as we gently build and nourish the body with new habits and foods.

In nutritional Strategy #8 I offer some important information about food sensitivities that can create problems with health and weight, but this strategy is only for those who are ready to eliminate a food for health reasons. If it is too triggering, help is offered to deal with the emotions related to this in the second part of this book. This is a fine line for many people; emotions are high when it comes to feeling deprived letting go of an allergenic food. If this is you, you are not alone. I recommend moving on with the last three strategies before trying to eliminate something in this way.

Is this list exhaustive?

Absolutely not—and I have purposefully kept it that way. I refer you to the Resources section for an exhaustive list of great nutritional and healing resources and information.

The reason for this is that I believe one of the biggest problems out there today is too much information and absolute overwhelm—which, frankly, is totally unnecessary. We are simply missing the target when we focus on each new and esoteric diet. I'm sorry, but it's just true. Are there fantastic diets from alkaline, raw, gut healing, and paleo?

Yes.

And guess what?

I've noticed my clients can't stick to them because of too many years of dieting and frustration. So this is what I have found truly works and gets folks back on the road to peace after years of struggle.

I'm not interested in throwing a lot of information at you that you won't use.

I'm keeping it simple, Goddess.

I've spent much time pondering what has to go in to these

strategies for results and what is safely left out for future exploration, and the first eight nutritional strategies in Part I are the ones I see as completely essential.

After so many years of dieting many people have lost track of any way of eating that makes sense for them and begin to be afraid of food.

I find, in giving my clients some very basic and simple eating strategies, they can get back into balance and begin to know the difference between an emotional craving and a physiological one.

Knowing the difference for yourself between an emotional craving and a physical one is *key* at this point in the game.

You can start with the food, or you can start with the emotions. If you are finding it too difficult to implement any of the food strategies, then skip right to working with the emotions and self-sabotage section of this book (Part II).

You may have heard some of the nutritional strategies before, and some maybe not. The goal is to have cravings disappear naturally when we eat what our body needs and balance blood sugar.

Though there is a lot of debate about how and what to eat, the simple strategies offered in this book are general enough that they can be applied to work for anyone to begin to heal from many years of chronic dieting and food cravings.

Most of all, every single one of these strategies is gathered from working with hundreds of women over the past eight years. This information is right from the street Goddess, not some book or fad diet. Sorry, that just doesn't work and it's why we all fail when we try it.

Any diet can work for a time, but only our bodies know what really works.

I recommend getting some healing around food by just eating sensibly using these eight nutritional strategies for a while without so much restriction. I don't recommend any one diet plan from vegan to paleo. I recommend listening to your own body's wisdom, and when you can't, be open to discovering it.

After all, the proof is in the pudding, right (pun intended)?

If you are feeling great on whatever diet you choose, great! Keep doing that. But if you aren't feeling great, then this is really for you. It was written for everyone who struggles navigating the diet and body image wars.

It's time to stop dieting and start living. Truly.

The last three strategies in Part II are essentially about healing the emotional reasons for not staying in action with health goals and implementing even the simplest food strategies. As I mentioned, you can start with either section, or bounce around using the healing work as you implement the food strategies for best results.

This advice is not a substitute for working with your medical or other healthcare provider. Please work with your healthcare provider ultimately when seeking to make changes with your health. It is highly recommended to get support from a qualified EFT (Emotional Freedom Techniques) practitioner for doing deeper emotional work if you feel stuck or overwhelmed at any time. Though the techniques can look simple and easy to use yourself, for true lasting results consult a qualified expert, especially for challenging personal issues.

Part I:
How to Eat Like a Goddess
(Instead of Being a Slave to Constant Dieting)

The First 8 Insider Strategies to Discover What to Eat and Why, from Your "Eat Like a Goddess" Mentor

Strategy #1: Hydrate

Strategy #2: Eat a protein breakfast

Strategy #3: Eat three meals per day

Strategy #4: Increase both raw and cooked vegetable intake

Strategy #5: Eat appropriate portion sizes

Strategy #6: Eat whole grains and legumes instead of processed as much as possible

Strategy #7: Know where your food comes from and eat organic produce and naturally raised animal foods

Strategy #8: Heal your digestion and food sensitivities that can cause weight-loss resistance (These are advanced health strategies, and it's highly recommended you work with an experienced integrative health professional to heal.)

"The wise man should consider that health is the greatest of human blessings. Let food be your medicine."
~ Hippocrates

"Those who think they have no time for healthy eating will sooner or later have to find time for illness."
~ Modified from Edward Stanley (1826–1893),
The Conduct of Life

"To eat is a necessity, but to eat intelligently is an art."
~ La Rochefoucauld

Strategy #1: Hydrate

Increase water intake early in the day upon first waking and hydrate throughout the day.

I'm sure you've heard by now that hydration is important to good health, but did you know that it can also assist you in losing weight? Water is absolutely critical to every cell in the body, and after a long night of rest the body needs to be hydrated. Drinking enough water first thing in the morning helps to move toxins and increase energy, to name just a few great benefits.

Make this a habit every morning and watch your energy increase and cravings decrease.

Another issue, and why we even need to talk about water, is that so many people are critically de-hydrated due to excess sugar in the diet taken in via sodas and other beverages that replace water, de-hydrating beverages like coffee, and/or some medications.

Yes, there is such a thing as too much water consumption, but your body actually has a thirst mechanism that, if you listen for it, will tell you when to drink water. There is also not really a "one size fits all" approach with water because if you are on medications that dehydrate you, working out and sweating a lot, or in a very hot climate, your water needs may be different.

One tip I think works well is to look at your urine. It should be very light yellow unless you are taking additional B vitamin supplements (which make the urine bright and dark).

Not all water is the same, of course, and water with the right pH, without added chlorine and fluoride and filtered to preserve mineral content, may be best for health. Resources to find filters or learn more are provided at the end of this book.

There is a caveat to hydration: Mineral balance is also an important part to proper hydration. This is a more complicated issue and something to be addressed further with an appropriate health practitioner of your choosing, but it is so important that it bears mention in any discussion about hydration. Important minerals that affect hydration are sodium, potassium, magnesium, and calcium. All of these are minerals that most people are significantly lacking in our culture today, perhaps except for sodium.

Did you know?

- While we can go for months without food, without water, merely days.

- Proper hydration is essential for optimal health.

- Our world has more toxins in the air, water, and food supply than ever before. *None* of us can escape this fact. Even polar bears in the artic are found to be excessively toxic. Our body wants to protect us from toxins and will store them in our fat cells. In fact, some excess weight may be due to toxicity. (For more information about how to gently detoxify the body naturally you can contact me at www.EatLikeAGodess.com.)

- Water helps to remove toxins from the body. The best solution to pollution is dilution.

- We can mistake thirst for hunger. A simple tip to decrease cravings may be just to stay hydrated. A University of Washington study showed that hunger pangs can be relieved by drinking one glass of water in 98% of the dieters surveyed.

- Up to 75% of Americans are dehydrated to the extent that it affects their health.

- The main cause of daytime fatigue is lack of water.

- As little as a 2% drop in the amount of water in your brain can cause confusion, short-term memory loss, and focus and memory problems.

- Water improves your skin, flushing out impurities and filling in the wrinkles, making you look younger.

- Water improves muscle tone. Muscles contract more easily when hydrated, making exercise more effective. Water flushes out lactic acid, preventing soreness.

- If your kidneys are water-deprived, the liver has to do their work along with its own. The extra work means it can't metabolize fat as well, and this sets you up to store fat.

Recipe for Success with This Strategy

Be proactive and prepared ahead of time.

1. Find several 24-ounce refillable water bottles. Stainless steel or glass is preferable for long-term use. (Plastic may be convenient, but it is not only filling our landfills excessively but our oceans as well. Many forms of plastic are also toxic to our bodies.) Fill one bottle at night and leave it beside your bed. Begin to drink it when you wake up and continue as you get ready for your day over the next hour.

2. Fill two more water bottles and have them where you will drink them throughout the day (maybe one in your car, one at work or at your desk, and another in your home).

Having water ready to go and on hand when you need it may sound like a simple thing to do, but it can help to create a habit of drinking enough water daily.

Strategy #2:
Eat a Protein Breakfast

Never skip your first meal of the day, no matter how tempting, and always include protein in it.

Hi, my name is Sandy, and I used to be a major meal skipper and breakfast hater! If you feel the same, you are in good company.

I understand that so many of us struggle with this important step. I get it. You are busy. You don't have time. You aren't even hungry. I know; I've been there. But guess what? Get over it! You are not going to create the changes in your health that you so desire without applying this most basic of food steps. It is, in fact, the very first food step to implement and maybe the most important of all.

What is most prevalent in our society today is skipping breakfast and even lunch, and eating most of the calories for the day at dinner and after.

I often describe this habit as the "upside-down pyramid" diet. We eat almost nothing early in the day, then eat excessively late in the day.

This is the number-one mistake you can make for your health and weight.

This simple habit alone will change your life. I have seen it over and over again. When it comes to how much protein and what kinds, we are all unique. The general rule of thumb to support a healthy metabolism and eliminate food and sugar cravings is to eat within an hour of waking and to increase protein slowly, adjusting for your own personal needs.

Let me explain why a protein breakfast is so important:

- Eating a protein breakfast within one hour of waking "sets" your blood sugar for the entire day.

- Skipping this meal can trigger stress hormones, which can increase blood sugar, which in turn triggers cravings.

- Energy crashes are frequently the result of eating a breakfast with too many carbohydrates and too little protein.

- A high-protein meal can increase metabolism by 30% for as long as 12 hours, the equivalent of a 3- to 4-mile jog.

- Animal protein includes a full spectrum of essential amino acids. Amino acids along with other nutrients are required to make important brain chemicals called neurotransmitters. Inability to make these important, "feel-good" neurotransmitters can trigger cravings (along with depressed mood and many other negative health consequences).

- Good luck fighting your own brain chemistry. Julia Ross, MA, in her book, *The Diet Cure,* describes these neurotransmitters and brain chemicals as being stronger than heroin. Your will-power doesn't stand a chance.

- We need a *daily* intake of complete protein to make these important brain chemicals that prevent cravings. Protein may be temporarily stored but is used quickly for bodily needs. All of your muscles and tissues require quality protein to build.

- Not all protein sources are created equal. Food combining to get your protein needs met, or eating nuts and seeds may leave you not only protein-deficient but imbalance your blood sugar. Vegetable sources of protein like legumes and grains have ratios of carbohydrate to protein that are just too high, and nuts and seeds have too high of a fat-to-protein ratio to use as protein sources on a long-term basis without health consequences. In fact, the only time I have ever seen anyone fail in my practice at kicking cravings or constant hunger is when they would *not* apply this one food rule correctly or consistently, and were stuck wanting to food combine. This includes me all through my 20s and into my early 30s. This mostly applies to my vegan or very food-restrictive vegetarian clients. A breakfast of grain with a nut butter is simply not going to provide the kind of protein required in my experience to end constant hunger and food cravings.

- People who skip breakfast or eat the wrong things at this meal, such as excessive carbohydrates, set themselves up for excessive nighttime cravings and out-of-control eating late in the day. *This habit alone contributes more to weight gain possibly than any other.*

- The excessive calories we eat at night will not only pack on extra weight, known as the "sumo wrestler diet" by Dr. Mark Hyman, but also ruin our appetite in the morning often setting us up for a vicious cycle.

Recipe for Success with This Strategy

1. Split your breakfast into two mini meals if need be. Make a smoothie or other breakfast and take it with you to

work. Have some before you leave home and some once you get to work.

2. Eat hypo-allergenic protein sources. Of course, anyone can be sensitive to any food, but generally speaking the top allergens for protein are cow dairy and soy. Try rice or other hypo-allergenic protein powders (there are now many on the market, as awareness of food sensitivity has increased), eggs, and other animal proteins for a cooked breakfast.

3. Make it easy to eat breakfast by shopping for foods for breakfast ahead of time, and have several options available. You can prep ahead with some things, too, like hard boiled eggs (a favorite breakfast of mine), or individual servings of frozen fruit in the freezer for smoothies.

4. We all have different needs for protein dependent upon activity levels and weight. I often recommend starting with a portion size the size and width of the palm of the hand to estimate. You will need to see how you feel. It may feel strange at first if you are not used to eating breakfast or a more filling one that includes protein. Start slowly and adjust as needed.

5. Give yourself time to incorporate new foods for breakfast and experiment.

Recommended Proteins

- Range organic animal proteins: bacon, turkey, chicken or pork sausages, eggs, smoked salmon, leftovers from the night before (one of my personal favorites), protein powders without added sugar of any kind.

Strategy #3:
Eat Three Meals per Day

Eat three meals a day, preferably within five hours of each other maximum.

Timing is everything with food. If you are eating your largest meal at the end of the day, as so many people do because they are so busy, skipping meals until the end of the day is a recipe for weight gain as you have already heard me talk about in the last strategy. Remember my example of the upside-down pyramid?

Though it may take time to incorporate this new habit of eating regular meals, for health and weight loss it is essential. I encourage you to figure out what works for you since we are all so different with our lifestyle, energy needs, and biochemistry.

For example, some people will eat two mini breakfasts as I mentioned, a medium portion for lunch, and a small portion for dinner. Others have a large breakfast, and a medium portion for lunch and dinner. This may sound confusing right now, but again, don't worry. The key point I want to get across here is to start eating regular meals within around five hours of each other at most to keep cravings away.

Eating a good breakfast and eating regular meals will help to stabilize blood sugar, which in turn may stabilize energy and mood, eliminate many food cravings, and help stabilize in the long term with weight.

For those of you who are currently struggling with blood sugar control, you may find that you need to snack between meals. If so try eating a small portion of a protein snack like nuts and seeds, hummus and celery sticks, cheese slices, sandwich meat slices, etc. You may find eventually that you do not need these snacks anymore as blood sugar stabilizes.

People who are also exempt from this rule are children, teens, bodybuilders, or other athletes who have a higher demand for calories.

Here is why eating three meals timed appropriately is so important:

- Snacking or grazing when not absolutely necessary (due to blood sugar control, health issues like diabetes or hypoglycemia or reactive hypoglycemia that can occur in adrenal exhaustion, for example) is counterproductive to being at a goal weight.

- We stimulate insulin every time we eat, and insulin is in charge of storing the calories from food we have eaten.

- Even low-calorie snacks can stimulate insulin release.

- We also inhibit fat burning in this way.

- Regular meals are required for stable blood sugar. And you already know from reading previous strategies the importance of stable blood sugar to your health and weight-loss goals.

Recipe for Success with This Strategy

1. The best tip I have to make this easy is to shop ahead for meals. If you like to cook, cook two days' meals ahead of time and bring them to work with you. If you don't like to cook, the same still applies except shop for prepared

meals you can bring with you to work or have in the house for a few days at a time.

2. Shop for only two or three days' worth of meals at a time. I think trying to meal plan for a week can get overwhelming. If it works for you, go for it. If not, just try having enough food on hand for a few days at a time. Make going to the grocery store a more regular habit in your daily life.

3. Have a stocked pantry so that all you pick up every few days are produce and meats.

4. Give yourself time to incorporate this habit. Be patient with yourself if this is new to you and difficult.

Strategy #4: Increase Both Raw and Cooked Vegetable Intake

Eat a wide spectrum of vegetables and some fruit according to individual needs.

As a general rule of thumb, eat six to nine servings of vegetables per day. If raw, a serving size is 1 cup, if cooked, ½ cup. I recommend going over this amount, but not going under for optimal health. Though there is a lot of variation to this according to your individual needs, climate, and season, this basic rule tends to be a big improvement for many.

An example of variation in needs is that when I am in the tropics I literally eat almost 100% raw vegetables and fruits, and very little cooked. It just feels natural and my body desires it. But in northern California, where I spend most of the year, I don't eat this way as it feels too "cooling" for me in this climate.

It is important to apply what feels right for us as individuals and our bodies at any given time.

Listen to your own body in this regard. If you feel good eating the way you are, great! If you don't, change something.

For example, I see so many of us living by what we think we

are supposed to be doing, like eating 100% raw vegetables. This was me when I first moved to the Bay Area from Hawaii.

Wrong! I was miserable. That just didn't work for me in my new climate. I also am a big proponent, not only as a chef and environmentalist but as someone who listens to my body and is present to its needs, of eating what is grown locally and seasonally.

Suddenly all of the tropical food just didn't appeal to me. It actually confused me at first, because I simply loved all of those foods, but I just didn't desire them in my new home.

It now feels totally natural to me that, without even knowing why, I just wanted to eat seasonally and locally. My body wanted to. My brain finally understood.

Here is why eating more vegetables and some fruit is essential to optimal health and weight loss:

- Vegetables and fruits have loads of vitamins, minerals, antioxidants, and phytonutrients that provide essential nutrition for the body, help to eliminate toxins and balance pH, and may be cancer preventative.

- Balanced pH in the body can contribute to weight loss and a better mood, just to name two benefits.

- Vegetables and fruits provide essential fiber, which is not only healthful to the bowel but helps to release toxins (which helps with weight loss).

- Vegetables and fruits have a broad spectrum of mineral content often. Increasing mineral content may help to reduce sugar cravings.

- Filling your plate and your stomach with vegetables at each meal tends to crowd out other, more fattening foods and contribute to weight loss. Calorie for calorie (though I don't believe in counting them) vegetables have much fewer than many other foods.

Recipe for Success with This Strategy

1. Add one new vegetable per week or every other week if you find eating veggies tough.

2. Eat raw cucumber, carrot, and/or celery sticks as snacks to get veggies into your day. You can even find them in just about any grocery store already cut up for you. No cooking, no prep, and lots of nutrients.

3. Find a green powder and use it daily if you can. There are an abundance of choices on the market. I prefer ones that are organic, low heat processed or freeze dried to preserve nutrients, and, most importantly, that have a broad spectrum of assorted vegetables in them.

4. Salads, soups, and stews are great, simple ways to incorporate more vegetables into your life. If you don't like to cook, learn one new thing per week or month if you can. If you buy already-prepared soups or stews add kale, Swiss chard, or other leafy greens to it to add nutrients.

5. Enjoy lettuce wraps. This is another great way to get more vegetables into your life and make a simple meal. Clean and prep romaine or other lettuce leaves ahead and have them ready in the fridge for a few days' worth of meals. You might add tuna salad, maybe some turkey slices or leftover roast chicken. For yummy additions you might add green onion, herbs, or whatever else you enjoy, and wrap it up as a snack or meal. I like adding a drizzle of salad dressing, hummus, pesto, spicy mustard, or other types of tasty sauces as well. Easy, fast and delicious!

6. Juice fresh vegetables and fruit. This is a fantastic way to eat more veggies. Find a juicer you like and will use regularly. My favorite, after using many different ones, is the Jack LaLanne juicer. It's affordable, easy to clean, and relatively small, and most important, the juice tastes

amazing. It changed my life with juicing, because it made it easier and tastier. That is just my opinion; see which juicer works for you. I've spent a small fortune on them and have ended up happiest with the Jack LaLanne. Best juicing veggie and fruit choices: beet, carrot, cucumber, celery, apple, lemon, kale, spinach, other greens you enjoy, ginger, turmeric (when you can find it; it looks a bit like ginger when fresh). I prefer using small amounts of the roots and fruits just for flavor, as they can have a lot of natural sugar. Also, leaving the skins on may add nutritional value, but be sure to use organic, non-waxed, or sprayed veggies and fruits for juicing.

Strategy #5: Eat Appropriate Portion Sizes

Eat slowly, and respect your individual needs.

What's an appropriate portion size?

Usually a lot less than we are used to being served so often in restaurants in the United States. I am not going to give you exact portion sizes, as that is very much like diet advice, and it doesn't really work in a "one size fits all" kind of way in my experience.

Different needs can be due to anything from athletic activity level, to caloric needs relative to different body sizes to individual health needs.

I will, however, give you some tips about how to get started knowing what portion size might be right for you.

But first, here is why eating the appropriate portion size is important for health and weight loss:

- You improve metabolic efficiency by not giving the body more fuel than it can use at any one time.

- Over-filling the stomach is a well-known stress inducer and there are implications on weight and health with inducing stress.

- Overeating habitually leads to insulin and leptin resistance, which leads to weight gain.

Recipe for Success with This Strategy

1. Try putting meals onto a salad plate or into a soup bowl so you don't over-fill a plate.

2. Substitute whole grains like brown rice, quinoa, millet, and legumes for processed white flour products and rice, etc. They are more filling, and we therefore tend to eat a lot less of them.

3. Incorporate the amounts given in the last chapter for vegetables into three meals each day. Remember: It is wise to go over the recommended amounts for vegetables, but probably very unwise to go under on a regular basis.

4. Do you eat and are still hungry?

   - Sometimes "hunger" is actually thirst. Ask yourself if you have been drinking enough water. Being hydrated early in the day (see Strategy # 1) and throughout the day will help with eating smaller portion sizes, too.

   - Sometimes, too, we may think hunger for more food is hunger for something besides a physiological need. Ask yourself if you are tired or upset, or need something else like comfort, relaxation, or reward. Begin to check in with yourself instead of eating. Is there some other way to fill that need? You can use the tools provided in Part II: Feel Like a Goddess to help you with the emotional need to eat when it persists. If you feel truly hungry, that's okay, too. Maybe you need to generally eat *more*.

   - If you are really and truly *physically* still hungry after one serving, you may need to notice if you ate enough protein during the day or in a meal, skipped a meal that day, or waited too long between meals.

- Another interesting reason for continued hunger that I have noticed after eating for many in our culture right now is due to leaving out an entire food group or essential nutrient. The three most common I see are fats of all kinds, from animal to vegetable fats, protein, and carbohydrates. Leave none of these out, and satiation is much higher in any given meal. The key is to eat healthful and non-processed versions of all three for best results with health.

5. Lastly, eat slowly. It takes up to 10 minutes for our brains to realize that we are full. Taste your food. Chew. Make mealtimes special. Enjoy them. Bring awareness to your mealtimes by turning off all technology like TV, phones, and computers, and take deep breaths if need be to stay present. Rushing through eating is a big no-no for weight loss and overeating, let alone for long-term health and happiness. Again, I think it is okay if this takes some time to really get the hang of. What's the rush?

Strategy #6:
Eat Whole Grains
and Legumes

Displace processed carbohydrates as much as possible.

Americans are eating more carbohydrates than ever in the form of processed foods like pastas, white-flour products, chips, and crackers, etc. The problem with this is that our bodies cannot metabolize that much carbohydrate. Processed carbohydrates like white flour enter the blood stream faster than whole grains. This causes an imbalance of insulin and therefore fat storage.

However, the opposite is not necessarily true that eating *no* carbohydrates is the answer.

We, as Americans, are a bit extreme. We go from one extreme to the other with our diets especially.

There were the all-protein/no-carb diet fads, which are still popular, as I write this, and many years ago there were high-carbohydrate/vegetarian types of diets that were popular and still are for many.

Either one may not be correct. We need carbs, and we need the right ones in the right amounts. Too much or too little are both problematic. We all need different amounts of carbohydrates and need to find what works for us as individuals.

The symptoms of not eating enough carbohydrates are just as serious as eating too many.

If you have been on a restricted carbohydrate diet for a long time, see if you can recognize yourself in any of these common symptoms of severe carbohydrate reduction:

- Dizziness

- Headaches

- Weakness

- Fatigue

- Nutrient deficiencies

- Nausea

- Diarrhea and digestive complaints

- Mental fatigue

- Bad breath

- Weight gain

- Not feeling satisfied after eating, or still hungry (Skipping *any* of the macronutrient food groups can cause this, by the way: fats, protein, or carbohydrates. Not eating enough of any one food group due to dieting is the most common reason for chronic hunger that I have seen.)

- Possible adrenal fatigue (This is from my own clinical experience.)

Why not start with eating small portions of whole grains (assuming no gluten sensitivity, which is discussed in Strategy #8) and legumes to replace the more processed varieties which can have less of an effect on blood sugar?

If we listen to our bodies, we can learn the signals that tell us how much is too much, or too little.

The bottom line for me has always been how someone feels, not what a book or even a great clinician teaches.

How do you really feel? Are you starving? Do you have constant cravings? Are you cranky or irritable, and do you have many health issues although you are eating a "healthy" diet? This was me many years ago, too. I get it.

It could be time to genuinely look at changing things up.

One sign that you might be eating *too many* carbohydrates is if you have cravings or are hungry after eating. If so, try decreasing carbohydrate intake and increasing protein just a small amount. Remember that too many carbohydrates, even in the form of whole grains, can contribute to blood sugar imbalance.

More reasons why whole grains and legumes may be important are that they:

- Contribute to a healthful diet by adding fiber, vitamins, and minerals, whereas processed grains have none, or have artificial additives.

- Can give energy if eaten in the right amounts for individual needs.

- Contribute to a feeling of fullness more readily and stop cravings for this reason, rather than contribute to them as processed carbohydrates do.

- Contribute to a feeling of satisfaction after eating and even fat-burning capacity.

Recipe for Success with This Strategy

1. Try one new whole-grain product per week, or per month if that feels overwhelming.

2. Find things that you love and don't force yourself to eat things you hate just because you think they will be good for you. For example, I will never like whole-grain pastas and I don't make myself eat them. I personally like adding

things like garbanzo beans to a spaghetti sauce and skip the pasta altogether. Works for me! Sometimes we have to think outside the box.

3. Read labels and recognize what is in a product. You may be surprised how much processed carbohydrate is actually in something. Awareness is key. This is a problem right now with all the gluten-free products out there. Many of these products are pure junk or filled with processed flour and sweeteners. Be careful with anything processed, even if you think it should be "good" for you.

4. Add legumes and whole grains to salads or soups. Throw some garbanzo, white, or kidney beans into your next salad or add whole-grain brown rice to a vegetable soup.

Strategy #7:
Know Where Your Food
Comes From

Eat organic produce and naturally raised animal foods.

Whether you believe there is additional nutritional value to organic products or not, chemical pesticides used to spray non-organic crops and other chemicals in non-organic food production have been demonstrated to be unhealthful *at best* for human consumption, let alone the environment.

These toxic chemicals may build up in our bodies if not released through normal detoxification pathways and contribute greatly to weight gain. Our fat cells store toxins to protect our vital organs.

Eliminating toxic chemicals in every way that you can in your life can only contribute to optimal health and even weight loss long-term. This includes those found in plastics, household cleaning products, makeup, and body products, as well as in the foods you eat. Your body will thank you and the Earth will, too.

This is long-term support for weight loss and general health that is so important, I had to include it in this book though you may or may not notice the results of a change to organic immediately.

Every step toward moving in this direction counts. You don't have to go 100% organic overnight, so please don't panic. Putting an end to the all-or-nothing, black-and-white thinking is a huge part of this transition into balance I feel for so many coming off the diet yo-yo in our culture today.

Every step you take counts, so never let overwhelm stop you from doing the small things that you can. Over time, it will all really add up.

Recipe for Success with This Strategy

1. Begin by noticing what you are buying and see if there is an organic alternative.

2. If you are eating approximately 20% organic produce now, shoot for 30 or 40% this month, for example.

3. Have fun with learning where your food comes from. Take a local farm tour if possible, or visit your local farmers market.

4. Grow your own herbs or foods as much as you can. Start with small planter boxes and grow as you can. It's fun, relatively easy, and very rewarding. At the very least those herbs sure smell good, right?

Strategy #8: Heal Your Digestion and Food Sensitivities That Cause Weight-Loss Resistance

(This is an advanced health strategy, and it's highly recommended you work with an experienced integrative health professional to heal.)

There is a lot of talk about food sensitivities and food allergy out there these days, and also a lot of confusion.

A true *food allergen* is the classic and immediate reaction that someone might have, say, to something like peanuts or shellfish that is unmistakable and very serious. The immune system has an immediate and acute response to a specific food or substance.

A *food sensitivity* is different. A food sensitivity is often a delayed reaction that can be unrecognized and mistaken for something else. The classic example is gluten sensitivity that can wreak havoc on the digestive tract for years without someone making a connection among skin problems, mood issues, and depression or digestive complaints connected to it.

For the purposes of this book, I'm not concerned with acute food allergens. These can be readily detected and are easily avoided because of this. It's food sensitivities that are a concern here with often unrecognized health consequences.

Why are we sensitive to a food, what can we do about it, and how is it connected to health and weight?

We often become sensitive to a particular food, or many different foods, due to a digestive tract that is not in optimal health or is "leaky." When the digestive tract, for various reasons, whether through overuse of antibiotics, poor diet, or stress, becomes "leaky" or out of balance in any way, we start to see many different food sensitivities.

A primary food sensitivity, however, is to gluten grains, which are prevalent in our society today. This alone can cause the gut damage in susceptible people to create the problem with other foods.

The true food sensitivity is often to the gluten grains, but people will become intolerant of many other foods later because of the effect gluten has on the gut lining.

Is the answer simply to remove the gluten, and then everything is better?

Not exactly. Due to the damage the grains cause to the cilia in the gut lining we have to repair that damage also in order for optimal health and healing to return.

The first step is removing the problem substances.

The next is healing the damage, and later restoring healthy gut bacteria and balance. It is a process and one worth doing.

One of the problems with food sensitivity is the frustration it can cause with weight issues. When the immune system is over-reactive for any reason, inflammation accumulates in the body and weight gain is often a result.

This kind of weight gain can make someone weight-loss resistant even while eating a whole-food, supposedly "healthy" diet.

What is healthy for one person may not be for another.

We are all unique. We have all experienced different stressors in our lives that contribute to this problem, and we all have unique genetic makeups.

I am focusing solely on the gluten grains here, as they are the predominant primary food sensitivity for so many people that create other food sensitivities down the road. However here are the top foods that people are sensitive to today:

- Gluten grains

- Cow dairy

- Corn

- Soy

- Eggs

- Artificial coloring and preservatives

- GMO foods

Do you notice anything about this list?

These are the very foods that most people eat *every day*.

By now you might be starting to see a connection here. If the immune system is reactive to a lot of foods it is because the digestive tract is not assimilating these foods properly perhaps due to a primary gluten intolerance.

If these are the very foods you eat every day, it makes a lot of sense that your immune system might have a reaction to them, right?

For many, a food-elimination diet is very illuminating. This is truly the gold standard, even above all the tests out there for food allergy and sensitivity. Your body doesn't lie.

If you do try a food-elimination diet, I highly recommend reading about it carefully first or working with a qualified practitioner, as it isn't as simple as it sounds to truly eliminate gluten, corn, soy, and dairy. These foods are often added to pretty much every processed food we purchase, from spice mixes to sandwich meats to sauces, and often people are unaware that the foods contain them.

The most important step is to understand the connection among mood, health, weight, and the foods we are eating.

Because the gluten grains are one of the most significant sensitivities out there creating problems with other foods, I want to give you more information about it here.

Also, in the Resources section, I list many great books that document and discuss this more thoroughly for you to check out, which I highly recommend you do. It's fascinating to discover that the sources of a lot of health issues can be cleared up with something so simple for so many! However, it is also a pretty big step to take for many to let go of old food habits and some of the grains that have been staples in their lives.

I get it.

It helps, however, to know what these grains may be doing to your health. Here are some of the most common symptoms of gluten intolerance:

- Depression, mood disorders, and anxiety
- Fatigue, foggy headedness
- ADHD-like behavior
- Abdominal pain, bloating, diarrhea, constipation
- Headaches
- Auto-immune diseases
- Bone or joint pain
- Low immunity
- Unexplained weight loss or weight gain
- Skin problems
- Hormonal imbalance
- Adrenal fatigue

One of my favorite teachers in holistic nutrition used to say this: "If your house was burning and your kids were inside, you would run in and retrieve them. No question, right?"

Well, this is your house burning, and what if a simple elimination could be an actual solution to some of your major health issues? And it's only a few weeks of your life to do a trial to find out?

What have you got to lose?

If you find out that you have *no* sensitivities, great! Now you know. Either way you win.

Recipe for Success with This Strategy

- Use EFT (Emotional Freedom Techniques) or Meridian Tapping for any feelings of deprivation that come up daily as you even think about doing a food elimination. (See Strategy #2 in Part II for more information about this part.)

- Get very familiar with common foods with gluten in them first before even considering doing an elimination. Many will eat gluten by accident, not realize it, and never discover the benefits of a gluten-free diet, while thinking they have actually tried it. This is a common roadblock.

- Do not worry about what anyone else is eating around you, looking silly, or being difficult or different. This is your health, and no one should be commenting on what you put in your mouth in my opinion. I highly recommend finding support around this final step, as many people find it helps significantly.

- Do not attempt to do a food elimination without working on food obsession or even food addiction first. For those struggling with food obsession, I recommend not attempting food elimination without working on the obsession first. I see this elimination backfire for many who feel they need the food for more emotional or stress related causes. For those of you who can relate, the next several strategies are for you!

Would you like support in implementing these strategies into your life?

Go to
www.EatLikeAGoddess.com
for your free audio training:

**How to End Food Obsession and
Love Yourself Skinny**

Part II: Feel Like a Goddess

The Last 3 Insider Strategies to Discover

How to Create a Winning Weight Loss Mindset & Lifestyle

Strategy #1: What a weight-loss mind-set is and why it is critical to your success

Strategy #2: How to let go of self-sabotage permanently, get un-stuck, and stop using willpower

Strategy #3. Create a lifestyle that supports you in your health goals (and why this is essential to long-term success)

"The only thing keeping you from getting what you want is the STORY you keep telling yourself about why you can't have it."
~ Tony Robbins

"Stop fixing your body. It was never broken."
~ Eve Ensler

Strategy #1:
What a Weight-Loss
Mind-Set Is
and Why it Is Critical
to Your Success

Find reasons why you can reach your goal instead of reasons why you can't.

*"Whether you think you can,
or you think you can't, you are right."*

~ Henry Ford

A weight-loss mind-set is created by setting an intention to achieve a goal, and then our actions and ability to actually achieve it. A good positive weight-loss mind-set is one where we find reasons why we *can* reach a goal instead of why we can't.

Resistance to getting started or getting into action can be because we have subconscious reasons *not* to reach our goal. This is when we sabotage ourselves and can't understand why we are doing it!

Let me explain.

An intention to lose weight may come from our conscious awareness.

We aren't happy when we look in the mirror or get dressed in the morning. We don't feel good in our bodies, have low energy, may even be having medical conditions that worry us, etc., so we want to change all of that.

A counter-intention may look like not wanting to exercise, eat vegetables or whatever we consider to be "healthy," drink more water, or having to stop eating junk food late at night or during the day, binge eating, or not making significant changes in our lifestyle to support our goal.

We have counter-intentions when we *know* what to do but can't get ourselves to even *want* to do it most of the time.

It shows up like this in many people's lives in the form of a lot of excuses why they *can't* do something instead of why they *can*:

- Not wanting to shop or meal plan at all

- Not wanting to cook but preferring to go through the drive-through for various reasons (mostly because of wanting the foods we are extremely addicted to)

- Not wanting to exercise and finding excuses why we can't

- Being resistant to change in any way when it comes to our habits or trying new things

- Having strong black-and-white thinking when it comes to food and having the feeling that "I can't eat anything!" (This is often far from the truth for so many of my clients but it can feel that way when someone has dieted for a long time and felt restricted. In fact, you can eat everything in the last section but probably don't want to, right? I get it.)

- Hating vegetables

- Hating any foods you perceive are good for you

There is no shame or blame in this, let me be clear.

It is simply that *something else that is outside of our conscious awareness* is at play often when this is going on.

A classic example of unconscious motivations that I see often is fear of *perceived* (whether real or un-real) negative consequences to achieving a goal of weight loss, such as: having to date again; attracting sexual attention; being visible; having to "get out there" in some way that feels threatening in general, including with professional goals; speaking up; feeling or experiencing difficult emotions; leaving a relationship; or changing something in their lives in a significant way.

My client "Rachel" is a classic example of someone with unconscious barriers to taking off weight. At first glance she just wasn't motivated to get into action and exercise, meal plan or shop, or eat healthfully. As we began to dig deeper under the surface, she uncovered a need to stay in a comfort zone for fear of becoming too sexy and wanting to leave a relationship that was difficult at the time we began working together. Ultimately she didn't need to leave her relationship, however, or stay in a comfort zone, but rather confront some old challenges and feelings that had gotten in the way of communicating her needs to her partner. By the time we were done working together not only had she taken off weight and felt motivated again with her health, but she had also rekindled romance and affection in the very relationship that she thought she needed to leave!

The weight can be a way to stay safe or hide in some subconscious way.

One of the best images to demonstrate this is the image I gave earlier of driving your car down the road with your foot on the gas and on the brake at the same time. The car ends up spinning out and going nowhere. We take two steps forward and two or three backward at the same time!

Again, I want to repeat: There is no shame or blame in this.

In fact, it is pretty normal for most of us at different times in our lives I think.

Resistance is normal and very common when moving toward goals for so many people. The key is to address it and not avoid it.

Resistance or subconscious counter-intentions are often operating when our motivation feels low, for example. When we have strong counter-intentions to achieving any goal we struggle to achieve it.

So how do we handle resistance, counter-intentions, or "self-sabotage" so we can take our foot off the brake and move freely down the road with ease instead of needing to use willpower or force?

In the rest of this section I will give you a few steps to get started doing this.

First: Recognize and identify subconscious counter-intentions to your goal with weight loss.

Here are more ways to recognize subconscious counter-intentions:

- You feel stuck, although you have tried everything to lose weight.

- You can't stop binge eating, or "emotional eating," though you are aware of doing it and have tried to stop.

- You eat secretly and furtively store food.

- You make plans to exercise but never get around to it.

- You find yourself making excuses about why you can't achieve your goal at times. When you start a plan to eat healthier or exercise, you find yourself saying things like "Yeah, but I can't do it because (name your reason)." Common reasons often sound like finding reasons why someone doesn't have enough time, money, or energy to do whatever it is they think they need to do (like meal preparation, planning, shopping, cooking, exercising, learning something new that they think they have to learn to do it, etc.).

Why Releasing Your Subconscious Counter-Intentions Is Critical to Successful Long-Term Weight Loss

Here is an exercise to begin to find subconscious counter-intentions with food and weight.

First, close your eyes and take a few slow deep breaths to get focused. Next, imagine yourself at your goal weight. Really try to imagine this. Who are you with? What are you doing? How do you feel? What are you wearing? What do you feel like at that weight?

If you have significant negative limiting beliefs or counter-intentions, you will not feel very motivated at best and totally defeated at worst as you imagine your goal or state it.

Here are some common negative counter-intentions that I hear often when someone is stuck with weight loss and tries the visualization above:

- "Yeah, but I can never stick to anything long enough to make it happen."
- "Yeah, but I won't have the time, energy, or money to do whatever I think I need to do."
- "Yeah, but I can't give up (name the thing you feel you will have to give up)."
- "Yeah, but I can't do it because I never have."
- "Yeah, but I'm too old/too sick/too whatever to do it."
- "Yeah, everyone else can do it, but for some reason but not me."

You get the idea, right? Are any of these limiting beliefs coming up for you as you feel into your goal?

If those beliefs are operating on a regular basis, day in and day out, you have a lot of resistance pulling on you as you are trying to drive down the weight-loss highway. When we have these kind of limiting beliefs or counter-intentions, we end up trying to use willpower and force often to achieve our goal, which usually fails eventually and leaves us feeling even worse than when we began!

Using willpower or force is never the best way to work toward a goal in the long run for ultimate success and happiness. It is why so many weight loss plans fail people over and over again.

You may lose some weight—maybe even a lot of weight—for months or even one year at a time, and then eventually it is all gained back and usually more in the end.

One of my clients, "Lisa," experienced this. She was doing so well with staying on track with her goals that one day she literally just woke up and scared herself. She was feeling so well, eating perfectly for her, and not experiencing cravings, and the weight was flying off. She went into a panic. But here is the catch: She didn't know why! So we applied tapping to uncover any hidden fears and comfort zones being triggered by her successes. When we tapped, sure enough very quickly an unconscious need to protect herself from attention from men came up. (This is an extremely common one for women, even if it is from something that happened 40 years prior.) For Lisa it was about fearing dating again and getting into a bad relationship if she lost the weight. She didn't even realize that would come up, but it did and at first it stopped her from staying on track. When we worked through it, she was right back on track with her health goals.

However, it was key for Lisa to be aware of what was coming up for her as she was losing the weight to stay successful with it. She had a lot of feelings about men that were in the way, ultimately, for her and that we worked to clear together. If she had not done this, the cravings I would bet would be right back for her as well as the weight "protecting" her from a perceived painful experience in dating.

It is a good goal to want to be healthy and achieve a healthy weight, but yo-yo-ing has damaging effects on our bodies and our minds. Avoid it if you can.

Releasing these negative subconscious limiting beliefs literally will release a significant amount of resistance to your goal and make the need to use willpower a thing of the past. There is some effort involved, but your efforts will often be greatly rewarded in having more peace with food and your body in the long run, which I think you will find is a true reward to your efforts.

Second: Release subconscious counter-intentions.

My favorite tool to find and release subconscious counter-intentions is to ask powerful questions. These questions often give us information that we hadn't realized before about how we are feeling and give us a new possibility therefore to release what holds us back.

Good questions to discover subconscious counter-intentions include:

1. Write your exact weight-loss goal clearly and specifically. You can state the amount of weight you want to lose, how you want to feel, and what your life will look like to you when you get there, for example. This is your conscious intention.

2. As soon as you state your goal, you may notice negative thoughts and feelings come up. These often take the form of "Yeah, but..." and may be significant internal blocks or obstacles to reaching your goal. Write down every negative belief that comes up as you think about your goal.

Common examples may take some form of the following:

- "Yeah, but I won't be able to maintain my weight loss, or all I have to do to get there."

- "I can't picture being at my goal weight. I have so far to go."
- "It will take too much work or be too hard."
- "I haven't been able to do it before, so why now?"
- "I'll feel deprived and like I have to eat foods I don't want to eat."
- "Even if I lose the weight I still won't be happy, so maybe it doesn't matter anyway."
- "I don't want to have to give up (name the food or habit)."
- "If I lose weight, others will be jealous or try to sabotage me."
- "I don't want to eat differently than (my spouse, my colleagues, my friends, my family, etc.)"

3. Address each limiting negative belief one at a time until they no longer feel so strong or true anymore. I use EFT (Emotional Freedom Techniques) for this, as it is the most powerful technique for creating change from within and releasing negative beliefs that I have ever used. In Strategy #2 I will show you how to get started using EFT. Using this unique tool you can get started accessing and releasing subconscious beliefs causing significant resistance to your goal.

Discovering what is going on under the surface may surprise you at first, but be excited because this is the first step to addressing it.

An interesting and often very unconscious belief that comes up for many women when wanting to lose weight and change anything in their diets is a fear of losing a partner or upsetting a partner who eats differently.

A client of mine recently realized she had often tried going gluten free, which was for her a very important thing to do to support her weight-loss goals, but she was secretly terrified of upsetting the status quo in her relationship. This was not conscious and was only discovered once we began tapping. Logically a lot of these trapped subconscious beliefs don't make sense to us, and for very good reason: They come from past experiences and do not relate to our lives now, yet they affect our lives until we release them, albeit without our even knowing it!

When we have so many negative beliefs about our goals, we tend not to even realize how resistant we are to achieving it. We've built up so much belief against ourselves that we have a hard time getting through the steps it takes to get there! This is why repeatedly stating affirmations doesn't work for many people. Their counter-intentions or negative subconscious beliefs are stronger than the new, positive intention they are setting.

Think about it for a moment. Do you start your day with a litany of negative beliefs about yourself, your body, and your ability to lose weight?

How motivating is that? Not very motivating, is it?

There is something you can do about it, however. You can begin to let go of all of the past beliefs keeping you stuck and not believing in yourself.

You see, your past is your past. We are often living today from everything that has happened in the past. But this moment is all we ever have to affect our lives. Every moment is a new opportunity for change if we let it be. Every challenge we face is truly an opportunity as well, but will we take it? That is the million-dollar question.

I'm going to show you a way to grab it by the *cojones,* my friends, and run with it so you can really effect change in your lives just like my clients do when they take action.

Here is a story one of my clients told me doing this process with her beliefs:

The voices urging me to eat all the time are gone...

Hi Sandy,

I have a peace inside me now that has been missing for years. The voices urging me to eat all the time are gone. This is such a wonderful feeling. Thank you for your help and I am looking forward to the next steps. I've lost 7 pounds and we have only just begun the program.

PG

PG had been struggling with those negative voices for her entire life, having no success in shifting her weight at all. She had tried many other great programs from Marianne Williamson's to Geneen Roth, diets and programs galore—you name it. Nothing had addressed the deeper underlying feelings and thoughts that were actually creating her sabotage.

For best results with the beliefs exercise you can keep coming back to it as needed as long as you would like in order to continue addressing negative counter-intentions getting in your way of achieving your goal of weight loss. I recommend taking any and all of them very seriously if you would like to get to the root of why you are stuck with weight loss.

Strategy #2: How to Let Go of Self-Sabotage Permanently, Get Un-Stuck, and Stop Using Willpower

Get your foot off the brake.

> *"EFT is at the forefront of the new healing movement."*
> ~ Candace Pert

> *"Our genes dance with our awareness. Our emotions and behavior have the power to shape our biology. This awareness can make a critical difference in health and longevity."*
> ~ Norman Shealy, MD, PhD

What is self-sabotage?

Why do we fail to do what we know we need to do to achieve a goal over and over again?

Are we lazy? Indifferent? Lacking in willpower?

Here is the thing: You are not lazy, lacking in willpower, or indifferent if you are still looking for answers and reading this book!

The problem—and why so many fantastic programs and even

diets fail so many people—is that we are looking in the wrong place for the answers to our problem perhaps.

We are shooting the arrow at the wrong target, and then thinking we have failed.

The answer is not in another diet when you struggle with getting into action. The answer is in *why* you don't want to get into action!

The answer absolutely must come from within and your own inner wisdom. You have all of the answers for you. Nobody else, only you.

I can just hear the complaints now:

"Oh great. If it's up to me I'll mess it up because I always have!" Right?

Wrong. If you've "messed it up" there has been a damn good reason, my Goddess friend. I guarantee it.

Here are some of the "good reasons" I've seen surface over the years:

- Extremely negative beliefs about food, their bodies, or weight that came from others around them, the society we live in, or from early childhood traumas or issues. We discussed negative beliefs about goals in the last chapter, and that is just the beginning for many.

- Emotional stress that overwhelmed them that is either conscious or unconscious that makes the food irresistible and an out-of-control urge instead of a choice.

- Nutritional deficiencies from years of low-calorie dieting, food restricting, stress, toxicity (which is just a part of what we all deal with every day on our planet today; nobody escapes this), and other factors that contribute to out-of-control cravings. You learned what to do to eat to fulfill general nutritional needs at this point in Part I of this book. If you find yourself unable to put the steps into action, all of the information in this part of the book is for you especially.

There is very good news of course on this front.

Through beginning to target where the real problem or issue is, as mentioned above, you *can* start to get real and lasting results.

When my client "Layla" started targeting the true causes of her weight, she began to get serious results and was able to give up calorie counting for the first time. When I started working with her she was addicted to drive-throughs, afternoon cookies, and late-night desserts of really any kind. She would get very sarcastic talking about those damn veggies, salads, and smoothies she thought she'd have to eat to get healthier and lose weight. She was cynical, pissed off, and frustrated with not just food but her life. With further examination it looked like there were many good reasons, too. It all seemed very logical. But when we tapped the true root causes of her current stress came up, which had to do with her past. This is very common, of course, with subconscious causes. It stems from unconscious stress and beliefs. Her current anger and frustration in her relationships was fueling her unhappiness and eating habits, but the current anger was not even current we discovered. It was related to her family of origin and very specific things that had happened long before. Releasing the past freed Layla up and for the first time in 20 years, without even thinking about it, she forgot to buy cookies or even go through her favorite drive-through—much to her surprise.

We tend to hold on to beliefs and stories from our pasts in very interesting ways, I have discovered, and just talking about it doesn't seem to help in changing our feelings about it. Tapping, however, has the ability to literally release the trapped emotion around an experience and allow us a whole new and better story. With Layla when we cleared the past she was able to literally stop eating the junk foods overnight. She didn't even think about it; she was just not doing it. I see this all of the time and it is what I call shooting at the *right* target: the emotions. This is when willpower becomes obsolete.

The tool that I use primarily with my clients to do this is EFT (Emotional Freedom Techniques).

EFT is a simple tool that you can learn to use to begin to release those negative beliefs, emotional stress, and cravings. EFT has been shown in research to significantly reduce and modulate the stress hormone cortisol.

Cortisol is a very important stress hormone that has gotten a lot of press over recent years. What people fail to understand sometimes is that cortisol needs to be in a very specific rhythm for our health, happiness, and weight to be balanced. It can be too high or too low. Either is very painful, and has specific symptoms and dramatic consequences for our health.

Releasing stress is absolutely key to maintaining a healthy weight and feeling relaxed, calm, peaceful and to balance cortisol. Imagine the power of having something that can give you that—and it is right in your own hands every single day.

Through tapping we can begin to not only release stress but the beliefs that hold us back. Emotional stress often creates trapped energy throughout our bodies that is the cause of much of our suffering. Releasing that trapped energy is the key to releasing the stress.

Many scientists, medical professionals, therapists, and healers from Deepak Chopra, MD, to Albert Szent-Gyorgi, Nobel Laureate in medicine, have discussed the power of energy in healing.

In fact, many now believe that the future of healing and medicine will be focused on how the energy field of the human body influences health and healing.

According to ancient Chinese medicine and Eastern philosophies, we have energy points throughout our bodies called meridians that can be stimulated to release energy and create balance throughout our bodies. If you have ever had acupuncture you understand this concept, except you have experienced this with the use of needles.

However, we can also gently tap these points with our fingertips to receive benefit with emotional release, as discovered in the last 20 years by two pioneering men, Roger Callahan, a psychologist, and Gary Craig, an engineer. (The full history of how these men discovered this can be found at EFTUniverse. com or at my website, EatLikeAGoddess.com.)

There are many wonderful tools for releasing energy or releasing blocks. I will introduce you to my favorite tool, one in which I have been an expert in over the years due to its efficacy in moving my clients and me forward toward winning not only the weight-loss mind-set game, but in reaching many other goals as well. This technique is EFT (Emotional Freedom Techniques).

EFT helps to access our subconscious awareness, which many people now believe is up to 90% of our actual awareness.

This means that we are often only aware *consciously* of 10% of what is going on at any given time!

What does this mean for our health and well-being? Well, I know from working with people over the years it can be the difference often between success or failure with many goals, not just weight loss.

Through tapping we can begin to peel back the layers to our core subconscious reasons for why we do what we do—even when we simply can't understand why—so that we can release them finally and move on!

People often ask me if they have to know all the hidden or buried beliefs in their subconscious mind. They fear that they can't access it if they don't know what it is.

That is the beauty of EFT. You do not have to know what the root cause is, and in fact how could you most of the time if it is "buried" in the subconscious?

EFT helps to bring it to the surface of our awareness and then release it.

Think of this process like bringing up something from the bottom of the ocean to the surface of the water. It is like a bubble that comes up, and then releases at the top into the air and is gone.

Here is a perfect example of how this works. My client "Barbara" came to a session so exhausted that she could hardly hold her head up and thought we might need to cancel the session. Since we had been working on both emotional stress and physical healing for her adrenal exhaustion I thought I would just check in first to see if it could be something physical. After we addressed all the common issues I quickly realized this didn't seem related to something physical at all but wondered if she had become emotionally triggered by anything in her life since she had been doing very well with her energy for weeks at that point. At first glance she said that nothing had happened, but when we began tapping for the fatigue almost out of nowhere something came up that to her seemed like nothing but that had completely tapped her energy level.

The interesting thing was that the event was actually nothing for her, but it had triggered a memory of something much more significant and her subconscious mind absolutely knew what it was related to. Within 20 minutes of tapping she had not only cleared that emotional trigger but completely regained her energy! It was quite astonishing to both of us, really, and a very quick and obvious result. She never again questioned whether subconscious trapped emotion could be a cause of her physical symptoms and reactions. In this case EFT very clearly brought up exactly what needed to come up to be cleared without Barbara needing to know what it was that needed clearing. This is common.

The process can feel therapeutic, but it is literally a release technique in my experience. Though our stories are fascinating and often incredibly important to whom we are, the beauty of this process is not in the story. The beauty of this process is in breaking free from the limitations that the story created from our past! The lessons learned remain, and we actually move forward into the present with true emotional freedom from the past, using EFT to release the trapped energies of emotion and beliefs.

Though skill and experience that are essential for getting the best results with this technique, many people can begin using it right away and receive benefit.

Please also understand that nuanced and advanced understanding of this technique is an art, not a science. Through certification and usage with myself and clients since 2003, I have become an EFT expert who is able to get to the root of the matter and get results faster. Though this technique will appear simple, and it is in effect, your results will be determined by understanding, knowledge, and experience, so give yourself time to practice for best effectiveness.

I always recommend working with an experienced practitioner for best results for two reasons. First, it is almost impossible to root out subconscious negative beliefs and blocks ourselves, even with experience. And second, an expert is that for a reason. An expert usually knows the terrain, what to look for, and common obstacles to getting there. Working with a professional or expert can be the difference between taking years to work on something (and most likely never achieving your goal, especially when it is something of this kind of sticky, subconscious nature) and taking weeks to months instead.

I say this from experience!

However, the simple tools offered in this book are enough to get you a quick start and a very targeted approach to healing.

Like anything, practice makes "perfect," and having a quick fix or rushed approach will yield spotty results at best. Having patience, consistent practice, and being focused and committed are the ways to get the best results over time in healing what is often a lifetime of living in a constant struggle with food and weight.

If it took a long time to get to where you are today, I highly recommend giving yourself the time it takes to begin to release whatever is in your way now.

You deserve it.

The Dalai Lama has said that compassion is love in action.

Give yourself the love you deserve and have compassion for yourself. All it takes is a moment to feel compassion and get into action, paying attention to your own needs. Giving ourselves kind attention, just as we would to others we care so much about like children or pets, is part of having compassion (and therefore love) for ourselves.

If you find it excruciatingly hard to find compassion for yourself and give yourself attention, I understand. This is extremely common. It is never too late to start giving ourselves the love we want, however. It only takes a moment. When you sit with yourself and do this work, you are doing just that.

What is offered here is a beginner's guide to getting started releasing emotions and negative beliefs that sabotage success.

Please note: By reading further and applying this technique, you are agreeing to take full responsibility for your own health and emotional well-being. If at any time while tapping you begin to feel uncomfortable, I recommend stopping and seeking qualified professional help.

How to Begin Using EFT (Emotional Freedom Techniques) to End Self-Sabotage

When using EFT there is a process that I recommend going through that we call "the basic recipe" for tapping. Is this the only way to tap? No. But when you are new to tapping, for best benefit you will want to use a map until you know the territory. That is my recommendation for best results as a beginner. I highly recommend having your "map" with you every time you tap and taking really good notes on specific feelings and beliefs that come up to be tapped on.

In my experience working with clients over the years, tapping is most effective when someone's intention is clear and focused, and a few other basic rules of tapping are met. The following are a few basic guidelines for best results with tapping.

How to Get the Most out of Tapping

1. Have an open mind, and be willing to experience something new and different, even if you do not understand it.

2. Be on target or be specific with what you are tapping on. This is one of the biggest issues that new tappers have. EFT works fastest and best on specific issues, so you will want to use the basic recipe until you feel confident in getting results for yourself. I always recommend working with an experienced practitioner for best results with tapping. Though it can look easy (and it is), there is a lot to moving through an issue and releasing it, and this takes experience and skill.

3. Be focused, turn off distractions, and really pay attention to your own awareness while tapping.

4. Be hydrated. You are moving energy through your body, and water is a conduit for energy. Being dehydrated can sabotage your results with tapping. Always drink water before, during, and after a session if needed.

5. Be patient with yourself and do not be in a rush! As you get better with tapping you may notice that you can tap for an issue and release it in a matter of minutes. In the beginning you may need more time. Anything worthwhile is worth taking the time to learn, I would argue, and tapping is no different.

6. Write down what you are working on. Get it out of your head and onto paper for focus and so you can see your own results. We often forget how much better we are doing once an issue is gone. It sounds impossible, I know, but it happens so frequently that it has a name in the healing world: the "apex effect."

7. Realize that you are accessing the subconscious mind
    when you tap. We may start with our conscious thoughts
    as we experience them, but where we end up comes from
    a deeper level of our awareness usually. I recommend not
    getting too attached to all of it or the story that arises.
    Being compassionate and non-attached is a great way to
    feel whatever comes up and let it go through tapping.

There are times when intense, unexpected emotions may
surface, and when you are new to this technique you want to
be aware of this. I recommend not going where you do not feel
comfortable going on your own. It is natural to need support,
and if at any time you feel that you do, please seek qualified
professional assistance.

As you use this technique you will begin to understand and
trust it more. Start gently and slowly. You cannot do it "wrong,"
though you will get better at releasing emotions and subconscious
beliefs with time, experience, and practice.

The "Basic Recipe" for EFT Tapping

1. Choose a specific issue or problem to treat for each session.
    Being as specific as possible will help with clearing it. In
    other words, if you can define the issue clearly, that is
    best. So if you are angry, you might describe the anger—
    at what or whom—instead of just saying "this anger."

2. Rate on a scale of 1 to 10 the intensity level or distress to
    you (10 being the highest).

3. Perform the set-up statement, or psychological reversal
    treatment by tapping on the karate chop point. The set-
    up or psychological reversal statement is not always
    necessary to use, but when it is, it is essential. For now,
    do not skip this step when you tap. The entire point
    of tapping with this statement is about releasing self-
    sabotage and this seems to have a very powerful effect
    with shifting it.

The reversal statement begins with the following affirmation:

"Even though I have this (state the specific problem, negative belief, or emotion), I deeply and completely accept myself and my feelings."

4. Tap through the meridian points with a "reminder phrase" of the problem. In other words, if the problem stated is anger or loneliness, the reminder phrase would be "this anger and loneliness" as you tap through the points. Keep it simple. When beginning to use EFT, keep it simple and it works just fine.

5. Generally we tap around five to seven times on each point with the fingertips. You can tap through several rounds of the points for an issue before re-assessing your intensity level. Using either hand or side of the body is fine.

The tapping points are: (See the picture of the tapping points on the following page.)

- Inside of eyebrows
- Sides of eyes
- Under eyes
- Under nose
- Chin
- Collarbone
- Under arm
- Head

6. If you notice as you are tapping that you no longer feel particularly lonely or angry, but now you are feeling frustrated (or whatever else comes up), stop tapping and *re-rate your intensity level with the original feelings.* If you can't seem to bring up anymore anger or loneliness, move on to the next thing that came up.

7. Try to stay with the specific emotions that you started with until they are at a 1 or 0 for best results. We can be in a hurry sometimes to move on to the next thing, but EFT will work best if you stick with one particular issue or feeling at a time. It may feel a bit funny at first to be so specific, but as you do this more it will begin to flow and make more sense. The biggest mistake new tappers make is *not* understanding this. We are peeling back layers and as it shifts you are clearing it. The key is to follow the threads and not stop right when you are making progress, and this can take some time to get good at following.

8. Take a deep breath and relax after several rounds of tapping before re-assessing your intensity level.

9. Assess your intensity level for the original concern. If there is some intensity level left, perform the set-up or psychological reversal again by tapping on the karate chop point and saying, ***"Even though I <u>still</u> have some of this problem, feeling, or negative belief (insert yours), I deeply and completely accept myself and my feelings."***

10. Tap through the points again saying, ***"This remaining (name the feeling)."*** You can tap several rounds until you feel some release.

11. Re-assess your intensity level. Repeat the above if necessary.

12. If you feel that you still have not been able to reduce your intensity level down below, say, 1 or 2, at this point a few things may be happening. The first is that psychological reversal is still strong. You can correct for this by doing the psychological reversal point again with feeling, and saying it several times. Another way to approach it is to ask yourself if you are ready to let this concern go. If not, tap for that. You might say, ***"Even though I am not sure I am***

ready to let go of this anger...." Another reason intensity levels may not go down is because we have switched to another aspect and didn't realize it. In other words, as mentioned earlier, be aware of what emotions and new thoughts are popping up. Maybe you have switched to frustration from anger or loneliness. Be aware of this and assess your rating on the original feeling. You may have completely cleared the anger. That is good. Just go on to the next thing.

13. Breathe deeply from your diaphragm after each round of tapping before assessing your intensity levels.

14. Be aware of what comes up for you in tapping. We are peeling back layers, and this often can bring up new thoughts and feelings. If you keep notes, you can come back to things to tap on them later and also track your own progress. **One of the interesting things about EFT is that as we clear issues, we tend to forget the associated feelings, once they've been cleared.**

15. So keep some notes and see how far you've come. It will encourage you to continue on your journey and heal more and more of what concerns you.

Prompt Sheet for EFT Basic Recipe

Tapping Points

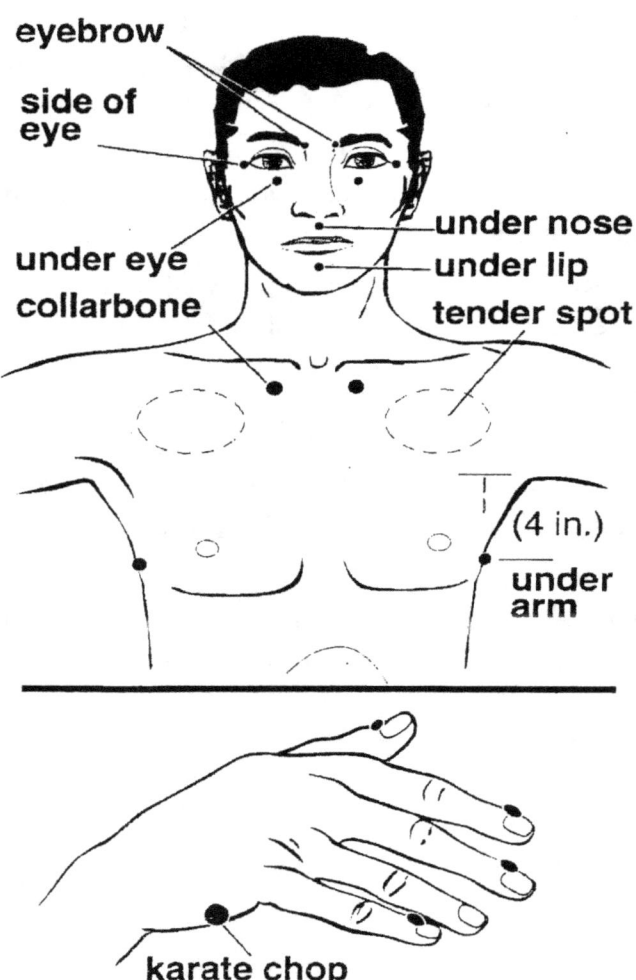

eyebrow

side of
eye

under nose

under eye

under lip

collarbone

tender spot

(4 in.)

under
arm

karate chop

Tap for Negative Beliefs about Food, Weight, and Your Body

Are you already overwhelmed?

If you are, then you have found an important place to begin to look to find relief with weight. But I think you will find as you get started and take it step-by-step, belief-by-belief, you will change your behaviors with food permanently instead of temporarily.

In the last chapter I gave a very simple but powerful exercise that you can keep going back to in order to find and release negative limiting beliefs.

I often just have people begin by tapping for the overwhelm they feel about this issue with food and weight in general because as long as we feel this way it is in the forefront of our minds, often distracting our focus on anything else.

Tapping for Overwhelm with Weight and Food

The first thing to know about tapping scripts is that they are simply a guide. The only reason I am giving you one is so you can have an example to follow or if you are new to this process. Please fill in your own feelings and thoughts for best effect.

Begin by tapping on the side of your hand or the "karate chop" point using the set-up statement.

You will repeat the set up statement three times on the side of your hand.

"Even though I feel overwhelmed and about this issue with food and weight because... (fill this in; one common example is this: I've failed over and over again in the past, and I'm not even sure where to begin. I love and accept myself, and I'm willing to believe in myself now)."

Tap the points using the reminder phrase or phrases based on the issue you are tapping for:

Inner eye: "I feel overwhelmed about the weight."

Outer eye: "I've failed so many times before."

Under the eye: "I've failed so many times. Why should this be different?"

Upper lip: "I don't believe I can do it."

Chin crease: "I don't believe in myself."

Collar bone: "I just don't believe I can do it."

Side of the body: "Why would it be different now?"

Top of the head: "I don't think I can do it."

Stop tapping after one round. Take a deep breath. Assess the intensity rating of this belief now. If it was a 10+ before tapping, has it reduced at all or has a new thought come up about this for you?

If there's no change, be sure to see if this is true. Do you suddenly feel like maybe it will be too hard and that is the real issue? Then realize you have shifted into another issue, and you no longer are addressing the original belief about your ability. This is where things get tricky for new tappers. Be sure you are still working on the same exact issue or belief.

If you feel no change at all even after looking at this, you can also be sure you are focused and hydrated, and try tapping for the issue again.

Keep tapping for several rounds to see if that belief begins to shift or release. If you feel it start to release I recommend tapping for some new possibilities or re-frames:

Inner eye: "Maybe it can be different this time."

Outer eye: "Why not?"

Under the eye: "I'm doing something different this time and addressing the cause."

Upper lip: "What if I can do it?"

Chin crease: "Maybe I can."

Collar bone: "Maybe it is possible if I am consistent with finding the underlying causes."

Side of the body: "I think it could be different now."

Top of the head: "I'm ready for it to be different now."

Stop tapping and assess your intensity rating on the original statement or belief. If it hasn't decreased at all, go back to the beginning and keep tapping. If it has but there is still some intensity, keep tapping until you feel the belief go down to a 0 or 1 of intensity.

At this point you can tap in the positive statement to really skyrocket your motivation.

Inner eye: "I'm willing to believe in myself now."

Outer eye: "I'm ready now."

Under eye: "I am able to do it now."

Upper lip: "I believe in myself now."

Chin crease: "I am completely committed now."

Collar bone: "I believe in myself and can do it now."

Side of the body: "I can do it."

Top of the head: "I am doing it."

When you finish these positive re-frames, assess how the overwhelm about weight loss feels to you. If you still feel significantly overwhelmed, I recommend staying with that feeling and tapping—asking why it is that you feel that way until you work through whatever fears and anxieties are lingering.

Often there is a strong desperation to lose weight because we think that we can't be happy until we do. I've discovered, however, that when there is an overwhelming strong desperation to lose weight for this reason, there is usually something else going on that the weight can easily be blamed for.

Weight can feel like the problem, but what if it is merely a symptom of another problem? When we heal that deeper "problem" or issue, the weight is no longer the urgent issue and tends to come off with ease, and in a gentle nurturing way instead of through the drastic measures I see a lot of people taking out there with food restriction, constant cleansing or fasts.

I am very fond of cleansing and detox plans for health reasons but I do not like to see people coming at this very healthful technique with the idea that they will go on them continually back-to-back as a desperate weight-loss strategy.

Cleansing and detox are wonderful strategies to improve over-all health and many will lose a few pounds during a cleanse or detox, it's true. The difference between doing them for health reasons or as a continual weight loss strategy is important I feel however.

In my practice (and in my life) I see people cleansing almost constantly as a weight loss strategy and this is absolutely detrimental to health in my opinion as it is a variation on severe food restriction. What is most important is the reason for doing the cleanse in the first place repeatedly and the reason is often desperation to lose weight.

When this is the case, I have found that healing the true causes of weight gain or the focus on the body as the problem in the first place must be healed for the weight to come off permanently.

Take my client "Lee" who lived on perpetual detox and cleanse plans that she had herself on every other month or more! This was her primary weight loss strategy. The only problem was; it didn't work! Worse, not only did it not work it left her feeling miserable, gaining even more weight, and with terrible food cravings and of course a total feeling of failure and no peace. She actually approached me at first to take her through a professional cleanse and detox for four weeks to lose weight. After I spoke with her I quickly realized the cleanses she had put herself on for a lifetime were clearly not the answer. When I began tapping with Lee, all of the causes to her food restriction and cleanse obsession came out and we were able to successfully clear them rather quickly. Like most of us, she had had several very painful experiences around body image so long ago in puberty that had actually created a whole belief system about herself. When we literally collapsed that emotional experience and the subsequent beliefs, she was free of the need to focus on her body as a "problem."

She was able to stop her obsession with cleansing totally. To my great joy and pride she began eating. Normally. Daily. No more "cleansing" which was really in fact starving herself. She stopped thinking about food. Her relationships eased. She wasn't so stressed over the holiday season even though she was with family where she normally would have eaten a lot more. That year she lost 8 pounds without even thinking about it instead! When I checked in with her many months later she was still feeling good and not obsessing.

You can't make this stuff up. It's crazy how powerful it is to just shoot the arrow at the right target!

The right target is almost always trapped emotion from painful experiences as well as the negative beliefs we create from those experiences that are out of our conscious awareness.

We live in a society today that has a stranglehold on body image, telling us there is one size that fits all.

We believe in good and bad foods.

We have extreme restriction and judgement about everything about ourselves.

I believe in taking a good look at how critically we are judging ourselves. Seeing how we make ourselves feel wrong, bad, and unattractive is an incredibly important step in healing body image for women in our culture today. What you are doing if you choose to do this work is healing for all of us. It matters. Your healing affects every woman around you, I would argue.

Let's all do the deeper work of loving ourselves and let go of this war we've created with food and our bodies once and for all, shall we?

You can begin by looking at the last chapter's exercise and applying EFT to the beliefs that you found there with your goals for weight loss.

Example of a Tapping Script for Negative Beliefs

Let's take, for example, negative beliefs about body image. I recommend going back in time to either the first or the worst time you can recall judging your body as wrong in some way. If you are like many of my clients, or like my client in the example above, the first or the worst time would be near puberty when girls often become body conscious.

This can be a fruitful place to tap to heal weight issues. However it can also bring up a lot of feelings that can be uncomfortable if you're not used to tapping. Again, I want to recommend if you ever feel uncomfortable while tapping, seek qualified support and help for best results. Begin by tapping on the side of your hand or the "karate chop" point using the set-up statement based on the issue (thought, feeling, belief, etc.) that you want to address.

Repeat the set-up statement three times on the side of your hand.

"Even though I don't believe I can lose weight because I've failed over and over again in the past, I love and accept myself and I'm willing to believe in myself now."

"Even though I have this memory of (insert your memory here) and for this reason I feel negative about the way I look, I love and accept myself."

Tap the points using the reminder phrase or phrases based on the issue you are tapping for:

Inner eye: "This memory surrounding (insert your memory)."

Outer eye: "I felt so embarrassed."

Under the eye: "I felt so ashamed."

Upper lip: "I felt different."

Chin crease: "I felt I didn't belong."

Collar bone: "I judge my body as wrong."

Side of the body: "All this judgment."

Top of the head: "All this shame."

Stop tapping after one round. Take a deep breath. Assess the intensity rating of this belief now. If it was a 10+ before tapping, has it reduced at all or a new thought come up about this for you?

If there's no change, be sure to see if this is true. Do you suddenly feel like maybe it will be too hard, and that is the real issue? Then realize you have shifted into another issue and you no longer are addressing the original belief about your ability. This is where things get tricky for new tappers. Be sure you are still working on the same exact issue or belief.

If there's no change at all even after looking at this, you can also be sure you are focused and hydrated.

Keep tapping for several rounds to see if that belief begins to shift. If you feel it start to I recommend tapping for some possibilities:

Inner eye: "What if I could let some of this go now?"

Outer eye: "Letting go of shame."

Under the eye: "Letting go of embarrassment."

Upper lip: "Loving the difference that I am."

Chin crease: "Accepting myself as I am."

Collar bone: "Choosing to see a new possibility from my current adult perspective."

Side of the body: "Maybe I was wrong then about the conclusions I made."

Top of the head: "There are many different shapes and sizes that are beautiful."

Stop tapping and assess your intensity rating on the original statement or belief. If it hasn't decreased at all, go back to the beginning and keep tapping. If it has but there is still some intensity, keep tapping until you feel the belief go down to a 0 or 1 of intensity.

At this point you can tap in the positive statement.

Inner eye: "I love my body now."

Outer eye: "I accept my body now."

Under eye: "I choose to accept."

Upper lip: "I am unique."

Chin crease: "I am beautiful as I am."

Collar bone: "What if there's never been anything to fix?"

Side of the body: "It's safe to stop fixing my body. It was never broken."

Top of the head: "I choose to love myself now as I am."

When you clear your negative body beliefs you also often become clear of food obsession and the constant need to fix yourself. Like my client Layla, this freedom is possible when a person does the work to clear the past beliefs.

Exercises to Find the Root Causes of Emotional Stress

Interestingly, when I work with people they are often not even aware of how much stress they are experiencing. It can be like the water we swim in: It is invisible to us sometimes.

A frog dropped into boiling water will attempt to jump out. But if you put the same frog in warm water and let it boil slowly over enough time, the frog will boil to death.

This is how we are with the stress in our lives.

Beginning to assess your current stress level so you can take a good look at it and do something about it is a great first step. Something often unknown to people is how stress from past events can also accumulate over time and cause significant problems.

The effect of this on food cravings is significant enough to cause a weight problem for many.

Here is just one example of how this can operate in someone's life: One of my clients was a working mom with two young children who simply could not understand why she couldn't lose weight or stick to any plan for long. She would always end up over-eating, binging on favorite foods, snacking on high-carb or sugary treats, and sabotaging herself. Food was her outlet for that stress.

When she began to work on the stress she was experiencing, however, what we discovered was that she felt overwhelmed, angry, frustrated, and fearful. She had difficulty in being able to speak up, set boundaries, and making herself a priority for many different reasons. This is extremely common for women, by the way, who use food when stressed. When we released that stress—not just discussed it, but *released* the beliefs and emotions involved—what do you think happened to her cravings?

Gone.

Yes, this took some work, but it didn't take years. It took a matter of several weeks of consistent, expertly-guided tapping and staying committed to herself and her needs.

Can you do that?

If so, you can have this freedom, too.

Finding the Significant Causes of Stress

Stress is something so many are experiencing on an ever-increasing scale, and stress can take many forms. We may be stressed about money, our jobs, relationships. We may even be eating and exercising in a way that actually increases our stress as well. Then there is the added stress of toxins in our water, air, and food that none of us can escape entirely.

Many of my clients report overwhelming fatigue and unexplained weight gain even though many of them feel that they are eating a relatively healthy diet, exercising, and doing everything "right." Few realize however that stress in any form, whether known or unknown, can cause weight gain.

Do you know what the major contributing causes of stress are that are making you fatigued, depressed, have food cravings and gain weight?

The most common contributors to stress are:

- *Unresolved* emotions, such as anger, fear, worry, anxiety, depression, guilt. (Interestingly, I have found that although many people have been in extensive therapy or programs, or have insight into the past emotional stress, it is still *unresolved*, which is of great significance to their health.)
- Overwork
- Physical and mental strain
- Excessive exercise
- Sleep deprivation
- Low blood sugar and poor diet
- Nutritional deficiencies
- Food reactions or sensitivities
- Toxicity

Here are some of the most common symptoms of severe stress or adrenal exhaustion:

- *Inability to lose weight even when exercising and eating well*
- Exhaustion not relieved by sleep
- Lightheaded when standing or sitting up too quickly
- Chronic allergies/sensitivities
- Cravings for salty foods
- Easily startled by noises
- Excessive anxiety or panic

Are you experiencing any of the above? If so, you may have stress-induced weight gain.

Some of the most common causes of stress, like sleep

deprivation, are obvious but what about unresolved emotions or food reactions, or even nutritional deficiencies?

Often, too, when we are under stress we do exactly the opposite of what our body needs to recover from it: We get less sleep and eat poorly because we are in a hurry. We start to take less time for ourselves, and many women start to eat less and exercise more as they see the pounds creep up. Though it can seem logical to do this, it's truly not a recipe for success with permanent weight loss.

We need to exercise to tolerance, not extremes. We need to eat more and better foods to support our taxed nervous system and stress hormones, not less. And we absolutely must get enough sleep to recover.

Here's why:

When we are experiencing stress from anything from the above list, our body releases an excess of stress hormones. At first, and for many years perhaps, we can sometimes sustain a high-stress hormone level and feel okay.

These same stress hormones can make us can also make us excessively excitable and anxious, and affect our sleep. Some people feel very productive at first but later, with enough time, cortisol will begin to decline if the chronic stress continues. This is when we are exhausted all of the time and begin to put on weight without even trying while we are doing everything else "right."

When cortisol is out of balance (either too high or too low), it can lead to out of control food cravings and weight gain.

Resolving Emotional Stress

The first step in resolving emotional stress in my experience is knowing where to look so assessing the above can go a long way in healing.

The next step, however, is just as critical: *releasing* the emotional stress, and of course making adjustments in diet, exercise, sleep, and other lifestyle changes that are needed.

Lifestyle changes in this way are a part of the process. Usually, however, when we begin by addressing the emotional stress in my experience, all of the other pieces seem to fall into place and become easier to implement.

In order to significantly reduce emotional stress, we need to find techniques that work for us and that we can implement quickly and frequently. Good stress-relief techniques are many and varied, from deep breathing, yoga, meditation, using affirmations and gratitude, to talk therapy.

However, none of these techniques offer the deeper healing and resolution that EFT (Emotional Freedom Techniques) provides, in my experience. When we work effectively with EFT we can uproot rather quickly and permanently in most cases the root causes for the stress. Often we can also make cognitive shifts and re-frame negative experiences in the process, giving us a more positive outlook for the future.

How does this work? I'll give you an example from a client to illustrate this.

I was working with a woman, "Sarah," to get un-stuck with weight loss. On the surface, all she knew was that she just wasn't motivated to do anything healthful from exercising to eating better. She knew what to do that worked for her, but couldn't get herself to do it. (This is such a common problem and always has a root in a subconscious cause, I believe.) She had out-of-control binges and was fatigued frequently. When we began to look at this issue, we were able through tapping (EFT—Emotional Freedom Techniques) and a process I use, to not only discover but release some major contributing causes for her. Afterward she was not only motivated to start exercising but found herself eating in the way she had wanted to for a long time, but couldn't before. All binges had stopped, even under what used to be stressful conditions, and she was happier and more energized than she had been in years.

So what did we do?

We found and released the major causes of stress for her that were actually hidden from her in her subconscious mind.

Healing the causes of a need to eat emotionally or binge, and the often-subsequent lack of ability to stick to a healthy plan of action, is truly possible if we shine the light in the right place, get the support needed, and allow ourselves the time to do the deeper healing we need to release both the past and the difficulties we face in the present.

Tapping for Emotional Stress

One of the most important things with tapping for emotional stress is knowing where to look. Here are some great questions to ask to discover current and past emotional stress and know what to tap for:

1. What happened the last time you lost weight? Was there a stressful event or several that occurred when the weight started to come on? (I know that after my mother died suddenly and unexpectedly, as well as several other major stressors happening at the same time, I went through major physical changes, including gaining weight. If you are gaining weight currently, what is going on in your life that feels stressful to you now? Is anything new going on? A new job, a new relationship, new habits, or a new living situation? Even positive things like a better job or new house you love can be stressors.

   Another way to ask this is: When did this problem begin? What was going on in your life then? Even bringing in seemingly positive things into your life such as a better job or a new house you love can be stressful. Common examples I see are loss of loved ones, loss of relationships, loss of jobs or income, getting inappropriate sexual attention that someone is uncomfortable with, body image issues that began as a pre-teen, and major life stressors of any kind. Some of my clients will tell me that it didn't begin anywhere—that they have always been this way. But try to recall the earliest time that you can when weight became an issue. Was it when you were 5? What was going on in your childhood?

2. Do you fear feeling deprived if you lose weight, or that you will have to be deprived of something? Are there emotional needs behind this feeling of deprivation? What do you feel deprived of? Ask yourself if you are feeling deprived of something in your life, perhaps (love, comfort, joy, support, fun, reward, peace, etc.).

3. Are there specific foods you feel deprived of that tend to be "trigger" foods for addictive eating? What time of day? When? Does it happen when you are tired or emotionally upset? Late at night?

4. If you can visualize yourself at your goal weight, how safe does that feel? If it doesn't feel safe, what about it isn't safe? Do you remember a time when it felt unsafe being thinner?

5. Ask "because" after you say a statement to get at a cause. Here's an example: It's not safe to get over this problem now because....

An example of safety was clearly illustrated by a client I was working with who was struggling with overeating. It took the form of binges, emotional eating, and being out of control with food at times. The effects in her life were wanting to hide, feeling depressed, and being unable to motivate herself at all to do much of anything to help herself. She didn't feel like exercising, doing activities she used to like, or sticking to any kind of healthful eating plan, which she knew all about.

What we discovered when we began tapping for her issues was that it *wasn't safe* for her to be attractive again because of something traumatic that had happened in the recent past—interestingly, right when she had started gaining weight.

6. What is the upside to keeping weight on? Or, what is the downside of losing weight? Maybe a downside is having to give up favorite foods or exercise, or feeling like you won't be able to enjoy social situations anymore or will have to eat differently from significant people in your life. Another downside can be feeling like you will lose your identity or something to focus on. The issue with food is very distracting. What is it that you might want to be distracted from? If you knew what it was, what would it be?

7. What are you feeling right before you want to over eat or binge? What emotions are you eating (stess, anxiety, overwhelm, fatigue, anger, frustration, loss, sadness etc.)?

Begin to tap for all of the above that are relevant for you using the basic tapping recipe you learned earlier. Give yourself the time, attention, and patience that you deserve to finally let go of whatever is really eating you, and in this way you will make dieting obsolete and your weight loss lasting instead of intermittent at best.

Example of a Tapping Script to Discover Emotional Stress

For finding significant causes of stress, you can start with some of the more general questions given above and start to peel back layers through tapping. One of the most powerful of all from the above questions is this:

What is the downside (or possible negative consequence) of taking off the weight right now?

Begin by tapping on the side of your hand or the "karate chop" point using the set up statement based on the issue (thought, feeling, belief, etc.) that you want to address.

Repeat the set-up statement three times on the side of your hand.

"Even though there could be a downside to losing weight right now, I love and accept myself."

Tap the points using the reminder phrase or phrases based on the issue you are tapping for:

Inner eye: "The possible downside to losing weight."

Outer eye: "I'm not sure there is one."

Under the eye: "If there were one it might be...." (Fill this in if you can.)

Upper lip: "Any possible downside to losing this weight."

Chin crease: "I'm open to knowing what it is."

Collar bone: "If I knew what it was it would be...." (Fill this in.)

Side of the body: "The negative consequence to losing this weight right now"

Top of the head: "Maybe I'm afraid I'd have to give up all my favorite foods and I don't want to do that right now because I need it for comfort (or any possible downside)."

Stop tapping after one round. Take a deep breath. Assess the intensity rating of this belief now or if something come up for you in that simple exercise.

If nothing came up, you might want to keep tapping and continue to ask the questions above as you tap. Even when we aren't aware of it there are often major consequences we fear for taking off weight. These unconscious causes are major saboteurs often to our goals.

Some common examples I see are fear of having to date, be sexual, or of getting attention from the opposite sex; fear of having to give up favorite foods that are needed for comfort, stress relief, relaxation, or other reasons; not knowing who you might be without the problem of weight and food; and avoidance or fear of moving forward in life or change.

We can start tapping for something rather non-specific, like there being a downside to taking off the weight, and get more specific through tapping. If you found something specific such as "I will have to give up all my favorite foods and I don't want to because I need them for … (xyz reason)," then begin tapping for that.

If there is no change at all even after looking at this, you can also be sure you are focused and hydrated. Then go back and keep tapping for several rounds to see if something might come up.

After tapping several rounds on the issue re-assess how you feel. Use this process repeatedly until you feel release from any of the stress that contributes to the weight gain and cravings you experience. I recommend watching what happens with the cravings and later with the weight as you tap.

The behavior with food and the weight itself are often symptoms of the deeper problem, which has its origins in the level of stress in someone's life, plus their negative beliefs. Continuing to tap daily for both is essential usually for many people when they begin this process.

The result is not just freedom from food cravings and lasting weight loss, but peace with food and their bodies.

Strategy #3:
Create a Lifestyle that Supports You
in Your Health Goals (and
Why This Is Essential to
Long-Term Success)

"It's not whether you get knocked down. It's whether you get up."
~ Vince Lombardi

"You, yourself, as much as anyone in the entire universe deserve your love and affection."
~ The Buddha

Creating a lifestyle that supports our health is also key to long-term weight loss. This can often make the difference between a quick fix that doesn't last and being able to sustain weight loss over time.

Life presents ups and downs and stress at times. It is not the stress or ups and downs that are often the problem, but our lack of capacity to deal with them—or our lack of healthier coping strategies than reaching for the food.

Having a lifestyle that is supportive of all of the nine previous strategies is especially important when the going gets rough.

When my mother passed away suddenly and unexpectedly in 2008, I became painfully aware of this need. I didn't realize it at the time, but I didn't have a solid lifestyle that supported me in long-term health and well-being. I was kind of flying by the seat of my pants with my "spirituality" and support practices.

Though I was lucky, relatively speaking, because I had all of the previous strategies to support me, as well as many others, I would have been spared tremendous pain I feel had I created more of a *lifestyle* that supported me.

I find this to be true, too, for all of my most successful clients. This is simply a strategy that cannot be skipped, and, frankly, may be most important of all.

Some of you already have this strategy down.

Congratulations! I salute you. You are way ahead of the game.

For those of you who could use a refresher course or need additional strategies for a lifestyle that supports you fully in creating the health that you want, this is for you.

Healthy Lifestyle Recipe for Success

1. **Create time and space for inspiration, renewal, stress reduction, and checking in with yourself daily.**

So often as women, we don't give as much to ourselves as we do to others. For men it can be a habit that doesn't come easily as well. And often in our busy lives we feel we can't take time for ourselves. We prioritize everyone else's needs over our own. We fill our schedules to over-flowing. We commit to things we don't want or need to do.

Yet, taking this time and space is one of the most powerful tools I know of in creating a healthy lifestyle. You can use this space and time to do some of the energy techniques and exercises that are given in this course, to meditate, to read inspirational books, to listen to meditative CDs, to write in a journal, to listen to music, or to do anything that feels rejuvenating. It is a time to check in with ourselves and go inward, and also relax and restore.

I recommend using the same space every time for the same purpose. Once you get used to using the same space, it becomes easier to use it for the same purpose over time. It becomes habitual. It doesn't matter if the space is just a favorite chair, a corner of a room with comfortable pillows, your bed, or an entire room, but be sure to find a place you love being in and can have time to yourself for anywhere from five to 30 minutes daily if you can. If you can't do it daily, try to make time for yourself in this way as often as you can.

Again, the amount of space is not the key here but rather the enjoyment of it. I lived in a studio apartment in San Francisco, and I still managed to find a corner where I could really be with myself that I enjoyed. I had a yoga hip opening chair that was my favorite chair and put it by my favorite window, and I embellished that corner with some favorite things that made me happy. It worked for me and it was very simple. You don't need a whole room; even a chair or pillow that you enjoy and will go back to repeatedly will do.

2. **Find simple ways to reduce stress _daily_.**

Here are some possibilities:

- Deep breathing. We can do this while we are working, in between activities, or before meditating or using other relaxation tools. Deep breathing is very effective at resetting our nervous system into a relaxation mode.

- Meditation. If you are new to meditating, try sitting in a quiet place for just a few minutes while staring at a candle flame. We don't have to sit for an hour necessarily to get to a place of relaxation. Make it easy for yourself; just do an amount of time that works for you and add more if you desire to.

- Epsom salt baths. Epsom salts have magnesium in

them, which help to soothe and relax our muscles and relieve stress.

- Nature walks, especially putting our feet barefoot on earth if we can. Being in nature is soothing and relaxing whether we are barefoot or not, of course, but being barefoot is uniquely grounding as we connect with the energy of the Earth in a way that so many of us are lacking in today's world.

- Use the space you created for inspiration and renewal to read inspirational books, listen to inspirational talks or other materials, or do any of the exercises given in this course or other healing techniques you enjoy daily.

- Restorative yoga poses. There are many restorative yoga poses. Find poses that work for you. Because we are all so unique and have different health challenges, it is important to honor where we are. I find using a pose at any point in the day, usually before bed, is extremely relaxing and restorative. A great book to begin to use some restorative poses is *Relax and Renew* by Judith Lasater.

- Exercise. What is the best form of exercise? The one you will do! Controversial I know, but it's just true. I don't believe that we all have to do the same form of exercise to see results. I do tend to lean toward a model that includes burst training combined with resistance and core training. That will get you fast results, it is true. But will you keep doing it? I don't know. If so, keep doing it. However, it is important to get our heart rates into the right zone for our age and relative fitness level in order to lose weight, get in shape, and stay in shape. I encourage you to follow appropriate heart-rate guidelines and work up if you are just starting an exercise program. Work with a qualified health practitioner if you have a health condition. But most importantly, find something you love doing and keep doing it! If you hate *all* exercise, you can tap for that feeling. Exercise is critical to good health, so find something that you will do. When you are enjoying exercise and not overdoing it, working within the right heart rate zone for the right amount of time for your own personal fitness level, exercise can be great for stress reduction, overall health, and weight loss.

3. Learn to say *no.*

Where have you said *yes* when you mean *no?* Do you feel pressured or too busy? Is there an activity you can say *no* to? The first thing most people tell me is that they feel guilty saying *no* to invitations or hosting others or to requests from family and friends. If this is you, try tapping to let go of guilt. Take your time and learn to say *no* if that feels right to you in some circumstances. Why do this? I have found that with women and weight especially, we are often suppressing our own feelings and needs. Anywhere we do this in our lives is extremely stressful, even if we aren't fully aware of it, and can contribute to a need to eat emotionally or binge. Even if this isn't happening for you, I believe there is benefit to addressing our own needs authentically in this way. Though it can be uncomfortable at first, often it gets easier and feels truly empowering with time. Saying *no* to something we don't want to do is saying *yes* to ourselves. Where can you say *yes* to *you* this week?

4. Be self-responsible.

Though being self-responsible is more of an attitude, I do think of it as a lifestyle enhancement that supports better health and especially helps with weight loss goals. Here's why: When we are able to take full responsibility for ourselves, we are often able to be more proactive and tend to feel empowered. How does this work? When we take responsibility for an action, behavior, feeling, or situation in our lives, we are likely looking for ways to improve or change it, and are therefore empowered instead of disempowered. When we are being self-responsible we realize the power is within us to change our situation to some degree, and we feel much more motivated to take action. We may not know exactly *what* to do, but we are willing to invest the time and energy into finding solutions instead of dwelling in the problem. It is an attitude that prevents the hopelessness that defines depression.

However, being self-responsible is not about trashing ourselves, being overly critical or blaming ourselves for everything that we think isn't working, or taking responsibility for everyone around us. It is merely knowing that ultimately we are responsible for ourselves, our actions, our beliefs and attitudes, and our own well-being. Even if we have been victimized by an experience in the past, it does not mean that we *are* victims. I believe there is a very significant difference, and in that difference is the key to either health or lack of well-being in the long run. It is our choice. I prefer to feel empowered. I have also noticed over the years that many people who are successful overall in achieving long-term health goals and weight loss specifically have this attitude. It simply works!

5. Get a good night's sleep.

Sleep is when we restore and there absolutely is *no* substitute for a good night's rest. Lack of sleep may contribute to an increase in stress hormones and blood sugar instability, which in turn may contribute to food cravings and weight gain. I could write an entire course on this topic alone, but to keep it simple, getting regular good sleep will change your life. I guarantee it. If insomnia is a problem for you I recommend seeking advice from your healthcare professional to help resolve this issue. In our culture today, however, making sleep a genuine priority is the most important first step. Turn off the TV. Turn off the computer. Even silence your cell phone! It's critical to health and long-term weight loss goals.

6. Be kind to yourself.

I can think of nothing more important to do than be kind to yourself. It's so easy to have a constant negative critique running in your head. Instead, be kind and loving toward yourself, your needs, and your process with healing and creating change. I see women on the entire spectrum with their relationship with food, from anorexic to chronic dieters to those with binge and emotional-eating behaviors. What do all seem to have in common? A constant dialogue of self-criticism. I'm sure this is not common just among those who diet or want to lose weight, of course, but whatever the reason it's self-defeating at best. It serves no positive purpose. Many tell me that they need to keep themselves in check with this criticism or that it is "just true" about them that they are bad in some way. If this is how you feel at times, I highly encourage you to be kind and loving to yourself always, no matter what. What would you say to a small child or your pet if they were struggling? Would you harshly criticize or berate them? Probably not, right? Then don't do it to yourself, either! Interrupt the pattern and affirm a new, more powerful belief every time you catch yourself going into self-criticism. One of the kindest things we can do for ourselves is tapping to let go of criticism.

7. Learn relaxation and stress relief techniques that work for you.

EFT tapping is one of my favorites and also one of the most effective tools I know.

8. Get support from a mentor, coach, or community leader whom you respect and trust when needed.

Getting support is a very healthy, proactive, and caring thing to do for ourselves. As women we are often quick to offer support to others but put our own self-care and nurturance on the backburner. I think that is the number-one cause of stress for many of the women ultimately that I work with: not prioritizing their own self-care. If this is you, I urge you to ask yourself why you feel you do that. For many there is a feeling of unworthiness at the root of this issue. We don't feel deserving of our own love and affection. And Goddess, you can tap for that! Please do it now. You matter. You do deserve it and you are worthy of your own love, affection, and care no matter what anyone else has ever said or done. Let that go now and use tapping if you feel stuck.

Tapping Script for Worth and Deserving to Prioritize Self-Care

Begin by tapping on the side of your hand or the "karate chop" point using the set-up statement based on the issue (thought, feeling, belief, etc.) that you want to address.

Repeat the set-up statement three times on the side of your hand.

"I don't feel like I can prioritize self-care right now because I'm not sure I should need all this time and attention and maybe I don't feel I even deserve it. That would be selfish...."

Tap the points using the reminder phrase or phrases based on the issue you are tapping for:

Inner eye: "I don't want to be selfish."

Outer eye: "Why do I even need to give myself that much time and attention?"

Under the eye: "I've got too much to do to do that."

Upper lip: "I shouldn't need that much time to myself."

Chin crease: "I can't prioritize myself."

Collar bone: "I have to prioritize everyone and everything else first. That's what I was taught or have always done."

Side of the body: "Sometimes I don't feel I deserve it."

Top of the head: "I don't think I deserve it or am worth spending that much time on."

Stop tapping after one round. Take a deep breath. Assess the intensity rating of the original belief now, or if something came up for you in that tapping round, tap for what came up.

This is just an example for one tapping round. The point when tapping is to feel the release of a belief or an emotion, and follow the threads of where it takes you. Tapping on self-care could lead to remembering a time when you felt like you always had to take care of someone in your family and were ignored, and you learned not to put your needs first. This would be very common, actually, to have something from the past come up, as I've mentioned before. Effective tapping involves following the thoughts and feelings where they lead in my experience.

I recommend keeping a journal while tapping, writing down the beliefs and emotions you are working on, giving them a rating. Keeping notes while tapping can help to stay on track if you are working on this alone.

Although putting into place effective strategies and lifestyle changes may feel challenging at first, it gets easier with time. Even implementing one strategy can be life changing. Remember, when I was in your shoes many years ago, I didn't know many of these strategies and their importance. Yet, I still was able to do it, and I know you can, too.

Words of Appreciation: Bringing it All Together

This book was written in appreciation for all the amazing and beautiful women I have known and worked with who have shown me that, truly, we are all goddesses and total healing of lifelong issues is in fact possible with the right direction and resources.

They have also taught me that "healing" is simply letting go of anything that is in our way, not something new to be created. It's like an emotional detox to get to the love and peace that are always our birthright and accessible under the storms of life.

All we have to do is shine the light in the right direction and stop our constant focus on food and beating ourselves up.

I have witnessed women who have struggled with extreme negative feelings about food, and their bodies let go of it in a matter of weeks (sometimes in merely a few short sessions with me) and it leaves me awestruck by what is truly possible and our creative capacity to change.

What once was a dark shadow in someone's life becomes a new opening for growth and dreams to emerge—often dreams they never even knew existed.

What holds us back with food also holds us back, it turns out, with our deepest soul purpose and happiness overall. And, by the way, this doesn't have to be a giant change, such as a new career. It could come through simplifying your life. The resulting success and happiness look different to all.

This is why I love doing this work.

People walk in the door thinking it is about food and weight. They go out the door knowing it is about love, joy, and purpose—and yes, feeling a bit lighter in every way, too!

Our darkest moments and biggest challenges are also our way toward the light and our biggest opportunities if we choose this.

My hope is that we choose the opportunity more often than the struggle, because life is ultimately waiting to be lived and enjoyed.

Healing Resources

Nutritional Resources:

For best drinking water I recommend Kangen Alkaline Water. This is a home water filtration device that not only takes out chemical compounds, and bacteria but also created alkaline water without adding minerals. If you want to know what true hydration feels like, try this water. I have used just about every water filtration system out there and never had this experience. Remember, thirst is often mistaken for hunger. Contact tapintohealth.com and tell them Sandy sent you for two free gallons of water if you are local.

Recommended Books: Nutrition

Ultra-Metabolism, **Mark Hyman, MD**

Sensible information about how to eat for health written by a very knowledgeable, holistic-minded MD. This is long-term, lifestyle nutrition information to be implemented for life, not just to get metabolism moving or as a hormone-balancing protocol.

The Hormone Re-Set Diet, **Sara Gottfried, MD**

Written for women who are starting to have hormonal symptoms to get back in balance and is more of a diet for this particular issue. It is such wonderful comprehensive and holistic-minded information from an MD that I'm sharing it here. However, my feeling is that this is a diet prescription for a particular issue and not a permanent way of eating after hormone balance is restored. Because hormone balance is a major issue of our times, this information is essential to understand.

The Fast Metabolism Diet, Haylie Pomroy

Those who have chronically dieted for too long, and even eating "sensibly" and not skipping meals or major food groups as discussed in my book, are still stuck with weight loss, could benefit greatly for a time incorporating some of Haylie Pomroy's strategies to get metabolism moving again.

The Diet Cure, Julia Ross

I can't speak highly enough about Julia's groundbreaking work. She is a psychologist who specializes in addiction recovery through nutrition and other means. She also breaks down body image so elegantly and powerfully. There is no such thing as a perfect size 2 or 4 or 6. (Each year the number goes down, by the way.) However, I warn against starting any supplement protocols in the book without expert support from an experienced practitioner. I have simply seen too many people get this wrong and feel even worse trying to be doctor and patient on themselves. This is not the fault of any of the protocols written in the book. It is simply that there is too much individual determination of needs when addressing addiction for any one supplement protocol to work in this way. It is why many of us make our entire careers about the nuances of helping people heal with nutrition, supplements, and emotional clearing work.

The Slow Down Diet: Eating for Pleasure, Energy and Weight Loss, Marc David

Re-gain pleasure with eating and drop the diet dogma that has created so much negativity around food. Marc is a phenomenal teacher about slowing down and enjoying food instead of the go-go-go, multitasking-while-eating culture we have created. Weight loss should be pleasurable. Don't think it can be? Read this book.

Real Food: What to Eat and Why, **Nina Planck**

Nina is heaven. I find this book to be so easy to read and understand and rebellious (as I am of course) about food and nutrition I can't say enough about it. Like me, Nina started out vegan and took the journey to whole foods and healing through whole fats and natural animal foods and products, and blossomed. She explains why we have lost our way in modern times and how to get back to nature and wholeness through real foods that our ancestors once ate for millennia. It's about our past healing our present fast food paradigm. She wrote the book I wanted to write 15 years ago. Now I just bow to her. Read it. It's lovely and healing for the soul.

Traditional Foods Are Your Best Medicine, **Ron Schmid, ND**

Ron is like the God of traditional foods to me. I used to keep this book by my bedside many years ago. I warn you: This is not for those who aren't truly interested in understanding our food paradigm of today. If you are not open to exploring something totally new and different (this described me once for most of my life, so I get it) then you may not want to pick up this book. If you want to understand how our ancestors ate for millennia before our modern food explosion, and decline into ill health and massive lack of well-being right along with it, buy this book. Read it several times. Do your own research and be amazed at how far we have come into "diet" nonsense in modern times.

The Gluten Connection, **Shari Leiberman**

This is hands down the best and most recommended book I have in my arsenal today on gluten sensitivity and what to do about it. She walks you through how to know if this is a problem for you, many case studies, how to shop and what to buy, and every single detail you would ever need to know about why grains are a current problem in our society. Most of all, it is very easy to read and understand and make use of immediately. The previous two books about traditional foods and traditional cooking methods also explain a lot about why we have so much gluten sensitivity in modern times so are worth understanding as well if this interests you.

The Yoga of Eating, Transcending Diets and Dogma to Nourish the Natural Self, Charles Eisenstein

This book changed my life many years ago and helped me to heal my own rigid diet dogma. Charles Eisenstein is literally a modern hero of mine. The title of the book says it all. I believe this book is very helpful for those who are feeling like crap while eating an extremely "healthy" diet and will not give up their rigid ideas of right and wrong with food. I see this often in vegans and vegetarians, which, as I said, was me once, too, so I get it. I will not beat around the bush: If you still feel like crap but are eating all organic, local, sprouted, "perfect food," there is simply something missing. This book could help you find it, Goddess. Don't wait; get it now.

Recommended Books: Energy, Psychology, and Healing

The Biology of Belief, Bruce Lipton

Bruce Lipton gives a scientific explanation of how our thoughts directly affect our cell activity. This book alone will change your life. I guarantee it.

Morphic Resonance: The Nature of Formative Causation, Rupert Sheldrake

Explains how past forms and behaviors of organisms determine those of similar organisms in the present through morphic resonance and reveals the nonmaterial connections that allow direct communication across time and space. Truly breathtaking work that I feel gives explanation to how we create as a group and as a culture, and why we are all a part of a much greater thought experiment than ourselves alone. The past is affecting us directly right now and we are affecting the future right now as a whole.

The Hidden Messages in Water, Masaru Emoto

If you've never heard of Masaru Emoto's work, it is truly one of the most profound examples of how thoughts and energy literally create reality. Masaru is a researcher who has spent many years cataloging the effect thoughts and sound have on water. It is truly remarkable and, I think, proof of our creative capacity. Speak highly of yourself and others in your own heart, Goddess. Your cells and theirs hear you.

E-Squared: Nine Do-it-Yourself Energy Experiments that Prove Your Thoughts Create Your Reality, **Pam Grout**

Pam is so fun it's simply a great read. She gives you powerful information to prove the point about energy and thought creating reality, but even more important, she helps someone to do little experiments that prove it to themselves. This is profoundly useful for anyone who just wants to believe and regain power in their own lives.

Waking the Tiger: Healing Trauma, **Peter A Levine**

Waking the Tiger offers a new and hopeful vision of trauma. It views the human animal as a unique being, endowed with an instinctual capacity. It asks and answers an intriguing question: Why are animals in the wild, though threatened routinely, rarely traumatized? By understanding the dynamics that make wild animals virtually immune to traumatic symptoms, the mystery of human trauma is revealed. This book is a must read for anyone serious about understanding PTSD.

A Course in Miracles, **Helen Shucman**

The definitive Course in Miracles text. I can't say enough about this book. Although the language can be heavily religious in tone, the material is non-denominational and timeless about love, forgiveness, and healing. Miracles are our birthright. We can make space for them by following the messages in this book.

Zero Limits, **Joe Vitale**

I have to admit that this is one of my favorite books that includes some of my favorite concepts ever. Maybe it is because Hawaii is like a home to me and I am a serious fan of Ho'oponopono, but whatever it is, I love this stuff. The concepts of love, forgiveness, gratitude, and ease, and joy with letting go are so powerful and will forever rule my thinking. Besides, Joe is just fun. Easy read. The book itself is a healing tool. Don't believe me? Check it out.

The Spontaneous Healing of Belief, Gregg Braden

Gregg is one of my favorite human beings speaking about change today. I can't get enough of him. I recently heard him speak about the urgency of getting together as a world community to work on climate change, and I was so moved by his combination of politics, social history and critique, and the power of healing that I could hardly speak after. He is right on in every way to me. He and Bruce Lipton are working together on getting the world community to listen to the power of our belief to create the kind of changes we need most to basically save our world from imminent environmental catastrophe if I understand correctly. In this book he gives detailed explanation about how belief is creative and breaks down how to make it real in our own lives. This book is an all-time favorite.

Power vs. Force, David R. Hawkins

About muscle testing, which is an energetic tool to assess unconscious knowledge and tap into precise answers when possible about choices we make. Muscle testing is a simple energy tool that I have used for more than 15 years and taught to clients to receive support with understanding beliefs and information that may be unconscious.

The Tapping Solution, Nick Ortner

An exploration of Meridian Tapping or Emotional Freedom Techniques, and an introduction to the use of tapping for beginners.

Courses by Sandy Available at DailyOm.com

Heal Subconscious Blocks to Weight Loss—8-Week Online Course to Conquer Negative Beliefs about Food and Body Image for Women

7 Secrets to Overcoming Food Obsession—A New Take on Letting go of an Old Habit

8 Secrets to Releasing Stubborn Weight—A Deep Dive into Emotional Healing for Hidden Stress with Audio Tapping and Scripts

Courses by Sandy Available at EatLikeAGoddess.Com

End Subconscious Blocks to Weight Loss—Home Study and Live Courses

Would you like support in implementing these strategies into your life?

Go to
www.EatLikeAGoddess.com
for your free audio training:

How to End Food Obsession and
Love Yourself Skinny

Get Your Free Companion Audio & Resource Guide Here!

"Insider Tips From Your Eat Like a Goddess Mentor: How to End Food Obsession & Love Yourself Skinny"

If you've struggled with diets that don't work, and you just want to love how you look in the mirror and feel like the goddess that you truly are and don't want to feel deprived to lose weight, I invite you to get your Eat Like a Goddess Support Package, featuring top-selling course author on the popular website Daily Om and chef to many high-profile celebrities and business leaders, Sandy Zeldes.

In this free audio program you will learn:

- **The Invisible Three**: Identify and release the three invisible barriers that keep you locked in a never-ending battle with food, weight, and your body.

- **Get Clear on the Cause**: Why weight is not the issue, food is not your enemy, and how to clear the root cause of those extra pounds.

- **A New Breakthrough!** A revolutionary process that makes is super-easy for you to clear hidden obstacles to losing weight.

- **Why Willpower Doesn't Work**: The real truth about willpower, dieting, and exercise, and why any kind of force or effort simply won't work.

- **The Deal Breaker**: The most important truth you must know if you are to ever change your relationship with food and your body.

- **Cut the Cravings**: The quickest way to retrain your brain so you no longer have the slightest craving or interest in certain foods.

- **Fall in Love**: How to relax into a sweet and loving relationship with your body and food, forever.

Don't Waste One More Second Obsessing About Food or Your Weight! You Know You Were Meant for So Much More!

No more diets. No more being jerked around by food or cravings. No more binge eating or reaching for those comfort foods any time you feel emotional or tired.

Stop wasting your precious time and energy focusing on food and your body weight! This is about you taking your life back so you can have more of who you really are, **more energy, more love, more joy.**

But best of all, you can release food obsession and lose weight with these tools with ***much less effort***!

Take the next step and sign up for your Eat Like a Goddess Support Package, a $97 value and yours FREE, my gift to you, full of rich information gathered over years of working with women to transform their relationship to food so that they can eat and feel like the goddess that they truly are.

Get Your Free Companion Audio & Resource Guide Here

www.EatLikeAGoddess.com